THE REAL
BEAUTY
BIBLE

THE REAL
BEAUTY
BIBLE

NAVIGATING
YOUR JOURNEY THROUGH
PLASTIC SURGERY

RICHARD J. BROWN MD

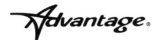

Published by Advantage, Charleston, South Carolina.
Member of Advantage Media Group.

ADVANTAGE is a registered trademark, and the Advantage colophon is a trademark of Advantage Media Group, Inc.

Printed in the United States of America.

10 9 8 7 6 5 4 3 2 1

ISBN: 978-1-59932-998-7
LCCN: 2019932030

Cover design by Carly Blake.
Layout design by Megan Elger.

This publication is designed to provide accurate and authoritative information in regard to the subject matter covered. It is sold with the understanding that the publisher is not engaged in rendering legal, accounting, or other professional services. If legal advice or other expert assistance is required, the services of a competent professional person should be sought.

Advantage Media Group is proud to be a part of the Tree Neutral® program. Tree Neutral offsets the number of trees consumed in the production and printing of this book by taking proactive steps such as planting trees in direct proportion to the number of trees used to print books. To learn more about Tree Neutral, please visit **www.treeneutral.com**.

Advantage Media Group is a publisher of business, self-improvement, and professional development books and online learning. We help entrepreneurs, business leaders, and professionals share their Stories, Passion, and Knowledge to help others Learn & Grow. Do you have a manuscript or book idea that you would like us to consider for publishing? Please visit **advantagefamily.com** or call **1.866.775.1696**.

Every journey in life requires the love and support of the most special people that surround them. When I decided to write this book, I knew it was going be a huge time commitment and stressful to my family's life. I knew deep in my heart that I needed to deliver this manuscript to the public because of my desire to inspire people to be the best version of themselves. I set out to help guide people to make the most informed decision possible when it comes to having plastic surgery treatment.

I grew up in Atlanta, Georgia and have two amazing, supportive parents in Bill and Rachel Brown. I owe this life to them and am so grateful for their support and belief in me. Without them, it would have been nearly insurmountable to achieve what I have so far. I have two older sisters, Tracey Appelbaum and Laurie Epstein, who are my friends and have always been there for me. I love you guys very much and am so honored and proud to be your brother.

I met my wife Alexis in 2004 when I was training in general surgery residency in Chicago. We then tackled our plastic surgery residency together in Nebraska. Being married to a surgeon in training is certainly a challenge due to the rigorous hours spent away from one another when being together was the most important factor for our development as a couple. She has been by my side for the past fourteen years and we have endured some difficult times and some exhilarating times together. She brought our two beautiful, identical twin boys, Brody and Grahm, into the world in 2009. They were diagnosed several years later with high functioning autistic spectrum disorder. Yet another challenge stood before us. Just like everything we have done in life together, we have tackled this journey with grace, love, and determination. The three of them are the greatest blessing in my life and I would give up everything today for them. I want them to know how grateful I am that they have allowed me this opportunity to express myself, and to help touch other people's lives in a positive way. I love you both more today than yesterday, but not nearly as much as tomorrow!

Love, your husband, best friend, and proudest father to Grahm and Brody Brown!

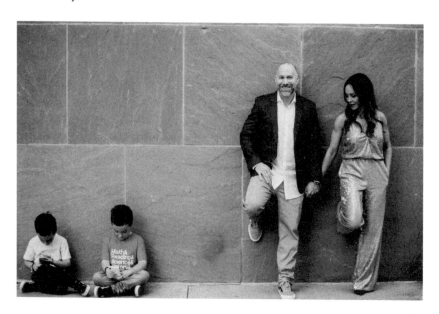

TABLE OF CONTENTS

FOREWORD

Toni Morrison once said, "If there's a book that you want to read, but it hasn't been written yet, then you must write it." And this, I suspect, is the impulse behind Dr. Richard J. Brown's book, *The Real Beauty Bible: Navigating Your Journey through Plastic Surgery.*

Having known Ricky since he was a clinical research fellow at Northwestern, I can tell you that all facets of his professional life as a doctor reflect the inner core of Ricky's being: he wants to help others. It's a mission that permeates the education of surgeons, but for Ricky specifically, this mantra is a sort of a fire that drives him as a human being as well.

With the thousands of patients Dr. Brown has helped through illness, disfigurement, and crises of self-confidence, I think he began to see that there were some common themes and patterns to patient questions and to his solace-rewarding answers. But as he looked through the available literature for patients and physicians alike, Ricky realized there was something missing. And as he did more and more research, he began to see an unmet need.

In typical Ricky Brown fashion, with the same dogged perseverance he applies to his patient care, Ricky started to collate and give substance to these questions and concerns patients had. But rather than make it an academic tome or something formulaic, Ricky stamped his written thoughts with a very grounded, almost folksy perspective so that in every word of this homespun book, you can hear Ricky's common sense and enlightenment in his voice.

The actual format of the book is itself an example of this as it is broken down in a very approachable structure:

Part 1: Taking the Leap to Regain Your Body and Change Your Life

Part 2: What You Need to Know About Popular Procedures

Part 3: Everything You Need to Know About Surgery— Before, During, and After

Dr. Brown distills the essential issues about patient engagement from questions about patient safety to indications for surgery, to operative detail, to postoperative management in a really accurate way. As a somewhat jaded and academically-imbued colleague, I find it rare to learn a significant amount from any one source but I really learned a lot about patient perspective and care from reading this book. The thoughtful manner in which Ricky put himself in his patient's stead not only makes for a commensurately thoughtful book but is an effective way to completely encircle patient education about plastic surgery.

Early in his book, Ricky depicts his own experience as a patient undergoing rhinoplasty surgery. Not many surgeons have that combination of empathy and patient experience and Dr. Brown is able to really bring credibility to his teachings because he always sees himself as a student of life first, and a teacher second. And listen when he says, "Having plastic surgery can be the best decision you've ever made—but it can also be the worst decision if you're doing it for the wrong reasons and don't choose the best surgeon you can find." This distills the essence of his book in a meaningful way and it really resonates with both patients and surgeons alike (it sure did with me).

There are so many beautifully written, simple, but resoundingly true aspects of this book that really cut through the fog of misinformation that sometimes surrounds plastic surgery. For instance, Ricky goes into detail about the issues related to scarring—a very common question both before and after plastic surgery. He rightfully notes that lasers and massage may help but that the majority of hotly marketed creams and topical medicines have a paucity of evidence backing them up (ironically Ricky and I collaborated on a research project looking at the impact of UV light on scar healing and we found that—contrary to common opinion—exposure to sunlight may actually help improve scars).

Another brilliant patient-centric adaptation Ricky writes about is how he uses a "vision board" to help manage expectations and get on the same page with his patients. I think Ricky's book is full of these succinct pearls to help patients understand the right surgery, find the right surgeon, and achieve the right result. Dr. Brown highlights that plastic surgery can make such a positive change in a patient's life—and more than any other book of its kind I've seen, *The Real Beauty Bible* shows you the way.

—John Y.S. Kim MD, MA, FACS

INTRODUCTION

Plastic surgery can be life changing for some people and life enhancing for others. I performed a breast augmentation and lift for a young woman in her late twenties who wanted the surgery so that she would feel more feminine. She also wanted to have breasts that fit her body, because she didn't feel like herself. She came back to me about five months later in tears, and I asked her what was wrong.

"Nothing's wrong, it's finally right!" she said. "You changed my life. I've never thought I could feel this way. I didn't ever think my husband would support me the way he did. I finally feel like who I should have been for my whole life."

Moments like that just make me pause and say, "Wow." All I did was give her implants, tighten up her breasts a little, and make them look pretty—and look at the effect it's had on her entire life.

If you're reading this book, you're probably considering plastic surgery or have already decided to have it. Maybe you're a mother or middle-aged woman who's lost her youthful body due to having children or because of previous obesity or maybe you have simply aged and are seeking body rejuvenation. Maybe you're someone who's fought and survived cancer, and now you want to put yourself back together the way you were before the disease struck—maybe even better. Perhaps you're a man who's thinking about some enhancements, but you're just not sure because, well, men don't do this, you're told. Whoever you are, you're interested, and you want to know more. Some of you are already confident, know what you want, and you don't care what other people think about your desire to have plastic surgery. You're in a good place in your life right now and want this for yourself, not for someone else. Those of you who aren't quite confident yet, and wonder what people will think, read on, because I can help you with those issues.

Deciding to have plastic surgery is a difficult decision. I know because I've been there (I had a rhinoplasty). But it's also a courageous decision, and it can be very liberating and empowering. I know it was for me. If you don't like some things about your body and want to change them, because doing so will make you feel confident and feel better in your clothes and in your skin, you can do it. You can have the procedure you want, rejuvenate your body, be confident again, and have a special, unique experience with your surgeon at the same time.

Plastic surgery is my passion, though not one that I realized until after I'd done many other things in my life. I once thought I might be an architect, because I enjoyed design and it intrigued me. My aesthetic sense might come from that.

I grew up in Atlanta and started college in Syracuse, New York, first majoring in communications. After two bitterly cold winters, I transferred to a school near home in Georgia (the University of Georgia, go Dawgs!) but didn't really know what I wanted to study. My dad started a company selling computers to medical practices, and I considered working in the family business. So I studied some business and economics, and I still wasn't sure what I wanted, but I knew one thing: economics was boring. I had to do something else.

I decided to take science and chemistry classes, and I enjoyed them and easily got As. I also decided to volunteer at the local hospital as a patient transporter who wheeled patients around the hospital. Things started to come together: being in the hospital environment and interacting with patients changed something in me. I'd never really thought about becoming a doctor until then. I realized that I loved taking care of people, and being in the hospital environment exposed me to everything about that. That's when I decided to go to medical school; I sat down one day, mapped it all out, drove home, and told my parents. My mom and dad were all for it and said they'd support me if that's what I wanted to do. "Go for it!" Mom said.

I put the pedal to the metal and took all my premed classes, finishing with a 3.8 GPA and getting into medical school in Chicago. But I couldn't start for a year, so I got a job as an orderly cleaning up operating rooms, and that's what got me interested in surgery. I started making friends with the surgeons, and I'd ask if I could watch them perform surgeries. One thing led to another, and my interests just kept growing. The more I watched surgeries, the more I wanted to become a surgeon.

My first contact with plastic surgery in a meaningful way was during my general surgery training in Chicago at an inner-city hospital. It was a knife-and-gun-club trauma center where we saw the worst of the worst cases. Stabbings and gunshot wounds to the belly needed plastic surgeons to close the tummies using reconstructive procedures, and it fascinated me. The plastic-surgery residents convinced me to go into the lab with them and do research, so I took a year off from my clinical duties to do landmark bench work and research on the topic of scarring and wound healing, and to write papers. Then I went back to my fourth year for general surgery.

That's when I transferred to Northwestern University, became certified in general surgery, and applied for plastic-surgery training, which was another two years beyond general surgery. When I saw how plastic surgery could transform peoples' lives, I felt empowered. The chance to have that effect on people exhilarated me, and I felt excited to have the honor and privilege of doing it. It was important to me to go all the way through and become certified in plastic surgery, a decision I've never regretted.

Now I get to take care of people from all walks of life and all ages—male, female, younger, older—and I can affect them and their lives in a way that I think few others can. I feel like I can help change peoples' lives, and it's a powerful feeling. When a patient says to me, "You changed my life," or "I'm a different person," that's the greatest satisfaction that I get from it. It's almost like when artists step back and look at their work, but it's really very humbling to me. I always see myself as that kid who was an okay student, who didn't crush it all the time academically at first, but who mastered something that he was really good at doing. I'm proud when patients are happy with what I've done to help them.

I love plastic surgery because the field is so broad. I can do a breast augmentation, but then right after that, I might do a breast cancer reconstruction, perform a reconstruction on someone's knee after an orthopedic procedure, or fix the aftermath of skin-cancer removal from someone's cheek. It's always something different. I've learned, too, that educating patients is a big part of what I do, and I love that part. It's a big reason why I wrote this book.

Having plastic surgery can be the best decision you've ever made—but it can also be the worst decision, if you're doing it for the wrong reasons and don't choose the best surgeon you can find. This book will help your decision to have surgery be the best one and, most importantly, it will help you avoid common mistakes that can affect you physically and emotionally. You'll learn about different plastic surgery procedures, how to choose a surgeon, and the entire process of having surgery from pre-op through the procedure and the postoperative process. To get the most out of this book, you should stay open-minded, be willing to hear the truth, and be okay with doing something for yourself, regardless of what anyone else thinks.

My hope is that this book will educate you, help you feel comfortable, and arm you with the knowledge and confidence to find a good surgeon and make good choices for yourself.

PART 1

Taking the Leap to Regain Your Body and Change Your Life

Having plastic surgery isn't about vanity. "I want this" is a legitimate reason for having a procedure. Maybe it wasn't in the 1980s or '90s, but it is now. It's okay for you to want a cosmetic or reconstructive procedure just because you want it, particularly if it's going to make you feel better. As a surgeon, I know I'm not just changing someone's physical aspects—I'm also helping his or her feelings of well-being.

What do you expect from plastic surgery? Are you doing it for the right reasons? What will your family think, and how will you tell them? These are some of the subjects I'll discuss in part 1. I'll examine two very important topics: finding the right surgeon for you, and the finances involved.

CHAPTER 1

When Is Surgery Right for You?

I ask all my patients an important question: Why do you want to have surgery? I want to know if they're doing it because *they* want it or because someone else wants them to have it. Patients absolutely must be having surgery for themselves and nobody else! A patient who says, "My husband wants me to have bigger breasts," or "My husband is really worried that my reduction will leave me too small," or "My wife thinks I'm too flabby," might want surgery for the wrong reasons. The bottom line is this: You should never have plastic surgery to please your partner, spouse, or friends who say you'd look better with a bigger butt, larger breasts, or a flatter tummy.

You have to understand your motivations for having surgery so you can make good decisions for yourself. I can relate to this personally, because I've been there myself. I had a rhinoplasty—a nose job. I remember not ever liking my nose and all the painful emotions that came with that. I'd broken my nose three times playing baseball when I was younger. I didn't feel ugly, but when I looked in the mirror, all I saw was my nose. I didn't know if I should do something about it, but it kept bugging me, and I knew nasal plastic surgery was an option, because more than one of my family members had had it.

I started to get serious about having surgery when I was transferring from Syracuse University to the University of Georgia. I remember struggling with a lot of emotions and wondering if it was the right time in my life to be having surgery.

I was only twenty-four then. I asked my mom, "Do you think I can get a rhinoplasty? Is it reasonable for me to do that? Am I being silly? Is this something I should do?"

My mom was pretty straightforward: "Yeah. If this is something that bothers you, you should do it. We'll help you do it."

So why did I want to have surgery? It was purely cosmetic. Period. I was honest with my family and myself about that. Transferring to a new school had nothing to do with it. I didn't pretend that I had breathing problems. I just didn't like what I saw when I looked in the mirror, and it really bothered me emotionally. I knew that surgery has risks, but I decided to do it, because I knew that I'd be totally miserable if I didn't.

In retrospect, I have to say that it was, no doubt, the best decision I've ever made in my life. Why? Because, afterward, when I looked in the mirror, I didn't see just my nose staring back at me. I didn't see any of the things that I'd told my surgeon I hated about my nose, and that was a very, very liberating thing for me. It gave me real confidence. Before, I felt like people looked at my nose all the time—they probably didn't, but I felt like it. Anytime I interacted with someone, I thought they were just staring at my ugly nose, and fixing my nose took all the noise out of my head that happened during those interactions. I finally felt like people were just talking to me, and that was a big deal for me.

I had surgery for me and no one else. I had it because I didn't like how my nose looked. What are your reasons for wanting surgery, and are they the right reasons or the wrong ones?

THE RIGHT REASONS TO HAVE SURGERY

- "I want my body back."
- "I want to feel empowered again in my life."
- "I want my clothes to fit better."
- "I want to feel better in my skin."
- "I want to feel like a woman."
- "I want my wife to be proud of how I look."
- "I want to look as good as I feel."

These are some of the things my patients say when they tell me why they want to have plastic surgery. Usually, patients can tell me very specific reasons why they want to have surgery, and that's an important prerequisite for surgery. You must know what you want and why, and the why has to be for the right reasons.

What makes a reason good or bad? Let's look at more good reasons for having plastic surgery: to restore youth, to fit better in your clothes, and to fix the aftermath of having kids (see chapter 9, The Mommy Makeover, which covers a group of procedures that women favor to fix their breasts, tummies, and other things because having kids wrecks them). Both women and men who've lost a significant amount of weight want plastic surgery to remove excess skin, and it totally changes their lives. They worked so hard to lose all that weight, and having surgery is the icing on the cake for them, an additional reward for their hard work.

These are all good reasons to have surgery, and people who want surgery for reasons like these should own those reasons. People who have surgery for the right reasons aren't trying to impress anyone, and they're not just trying to look hot in an outfit. They're trying to feel like themselves in their clothing—feel comfortable in their own skin again. They want to own their bodies again.

I take time to understand a patient's reasons and motives for having surgery to make sure it's a good decision for both of us. I don't want to do a procedure on someone who wants it for the wrong reasons. Suppose a patient says to me, "My husband wants me to have breast augmentation."

I'd look her straight the eyes and say, "What do *you* want?" If she can't answer that question, I'd tell her that we'll talk about the operation, but she needs to come back with the reasons why she wants it, what she thinks it's going to do for her, and how it's going to bring back into her life whatever it is she thinks she's missing. I need to know her real, honest reasons, because they're so important to the surgery's long-term success.

Good reasons for having surgery aren't all purely cosmetic. People have plastic surgery to correct deformities, repair tissue damage from an injury, improve breathing, or to enhance a feature that didn't develop properly. Breast cancer patients might want reconstructive surgery to feel feminine or whole again. Battered patients—women or men—can have surgery to revise scars, which can change their lives because it can erase the physical memory of what happened and allow them to move on from their trauma.

I'm particularly passionate about doing breast reduction surgery to help over-endowed teenagers—both boys and girls—who are teased and bullied. Reduction surgery can be truly life changing for them. I've seen fourteen-year old girls with breasts literally as large as my head (it's a genetic thing). People stared and laughed at them, and physical education class in school was just unbearable for them, because they couldn't take part in some of the activities. They're so happy after reduction surgery, and I love seeing that. One fifteen-year-old boy with gynecomastia ("man boobs") couldn't take his shirt off in the school locker room, and the external embarrassment he suffered from the kids' teasing was nothing compared with his inner embarrassment. He was introverted, shy, and had no energy. I lipo-suctioned the breasts, took out some of the fibrous tissue, and put him into chest compression for six weeks. When he came back for his follow-up appointment, he'd changed completely. Now he was an outgoing, engaged, energetic kid—a different child entirely. Helping kids like these is so satisfying for me, because their mental well-being is so important, and I truly believe these surgeries can often change the course of their lives.

THE WRONG REASONS TO HAVE SURGERY

I sometimes turn patients away because their reasons for wanting surgery are the wrong reasons. I mentioned some of the wrong reasons already, but they're worth repeating in the following list, because the consequences of having surgery for the wrong reasons are just too great.

- **Unrealistic expectations.** Patients might think that having surgery will keep a marriage from falling apart, help them find a new partner, or make them popular, but none of those reasons are realistic.

- **Doing it for someone else (husband, wife, or partner).** It's possible the patient could regret his or her decision when it's too late and face psychological impacts. The patient is the only person whose wants matter.

- **Obsession with perfection.** A patient who's had multiple surgeries can become so obsessed with the idea of imperfection that a happy surgical result might never be possible.

- **The wrong time in the patient's life.** For example, the patient might really want her breasts to look more rejuvenated, but she also wants to have more children. Maybe she wants the perfect tummy tuck, but she needs to lose twenty pounds first.

- **Trying to impress others or gain social acceptance.** As with having surgery for a spouse or partner, doing so to impress friends or social groups in hopes of being more popular carries the same risks of regret and psychological impacts.

- **Doing it to "start over."** Sometimes patients think surgery will be a new beginning after a divorce. I always tread lightly when this comes up. I usually ask if they would still want surgery if they weren't getting divorced, and sometimes they say no, they wouldn't want it.

If I think a patient wants a procedure for the wrong reasons, we'll have a serious, straightforward talk. A young mother who wants a breast augmentation and still wants to have more kids afterward, for example, would spend all that money for surgery and possibly ruin the results after having more children. For someone like her, it isn't the right time for the procedure, and if she can just wait until after she has her kids, she can come back and do it. (That said, I think breast augmentation or surgery is okay for a woman in her twenties who won't be having kids for ten years or so.) Similarly, a woman who wants a tummy tuck but still needs to lose twenty pounds will waste her money because she'd need another tuck after she lost the weight. Timing can be everything. I sometimes risk losing such patients because of their right-now attitude and inability to understand that they need to do what I recommend if they want long-term happiness and the best result possible.

Do you know if this is a good time for you to have your procedure? Do you know why you want it? Have you even thought about these things? You probably need to ask yourself these questions.

Remember, your motives for having surgery should be your own—totally. You don't do it so that you can be a better model. You don't do it because all your friends are doing it and insist that you should, too. You don't do it to impress your husband or wife, your boss, or your social groups. And you *especially* don't do because you think that if you look as attractive as other men or women do, your spouse won't want

Self-Assessment: Ten Questions to Ask Yourself

1. Why do I want this surgery?
2. Am I doing this for myself or for someone else?
3. Do I know and accept the risks involved?
4. What are my expectations from the surgery?
5. What will I do if the results aren't what I expect?
6. Is this the best time for me to have this surgery?
7. Am I ready for this surgery emotionally?
8. Do I have support from others in my life?
9. Can I afford this surgery?
10. Am I worried about what others will think if I have surgery?

to leave you, and you'll save your marriage. Those are *not* the right reasons. You have to do it 100 percent for yourself.

SURGERY RISKS

Any surgery comes with risks, and anyone considering plastic surgery has to know and understand those risks and accept them before having the procedure. General risks that come with any surgery include, but aren't limited to, the following:

- Delayed wound healing

- Bleeding (hematoma)

- Fluid collection (seroma)

- Infections

- Poor scarring

- Discomfort

- Asymmetry

- Decreased skin sensation

- Contour irregularities

- Bruising and swelling

- Skin sensitivity

- A need for additional procedures

Your surgeon will discuss the risks involved in any procedure that you're considering. Make sure you listen carefully and understand everything you're told, and if you don't understand something or need more information, please ask.

SCARS

If you want plastic surgery, you have to accept the scars that come with it or the procedure won't be worth it. Scars are unavoidable, and there's no such thing as scarless surgery (though as a plastic surgeon, I feel that I can create much prettier scars than anyone else can because of my training). The tendency to scar can be genetic—patients of certain ethnicities tend to form thicker, darker scars. Some people are genetically disposed to forming raised scars (hypertrophic) or excessive growth of scar tissue (keloids). I sometimes ask patients to show me scars on their bodies so I can assess their scarring tendencies and can prepare them for how their scars might look. The least aesthetic scars tend to form over areas of greater tension, such as joints, extremities, and on the back. Again, scarless surgery doesn't exist, but we have therapies that will help reduce scar appearance and improve quality. Silicone scar therapy started two to three weeks after surgery is one of the best treatments proven in the literature to work to reduce the scar's redness and decrease its thickness. Sometimes laser therapy can help to fade scars or reduce their thickness. I teach patients how to massage their scars daily for many months. It's a form of pressure therapy proven in the medical literature to help improve scars' quality and appearance. The literature has not shown that scar creams, vitamin E, and other treatments that patients ask me about can improve scarring.[1]

You shouldn't have any plastic surgery procedure if you're not willing to accept the scars that come with it. Some of my patients reconsidered surgery after I discussed all of the incisions I'd be making. They realized they didn't want all those scars and thought, "Maybe this isn't for me." And they didn't do it. It's uncommon, but some people decide it's not for them because of the scarring.

---

1   Volkan Tanaydin et al., "The Role of Topical Vitamin E in Scar Management: A Systematic Review," *Aesthetic Surgery Journal 36, no. 8 (2016): 959–65, https://doi.org/10.1093/asj/sjw046.*

CHAPTER 2

Expectations — What You
Want and What's Possible

One of the most important things I do with new patients is sort through their expectations and try to manage them. Patients considering plastic surgery can be all over the place about what they want, what they expect a surgeon can do, and what's actually possible. Others know exactly what they want and are open to hearing about what's realistic. The surgeon and the patient have to agree on what's realistic or the patient won't be happy with the results.

Some patients are far too optimistic about what surgery can accomplish. Ideal patients know what they want, which means they also know what they don't like about their bodies and can be quite specific when describing their dislikes. Sometimes they know, but they just don't articulate it well. Because the consultation's goal is to provide the surgeon with the information needed to determine realistic goals, patients who can't be specific about their wants and expectations make it hard for their surgeon to deliver satisfying results.

KNOWING WHAT YOU WANT AND GETTING WHAT YOU WANT

Very early in my career, I had a patient—a woman in her thirties—who had a breast reduction, and then she went on to have children. Afterward, her breasts got smaller and were a little flat on top, so then she wanted an augmentation. We talked a lot about what she wanted, such as breast size, how she wanted them to look, the different types of implants, and what the implants could and couldn't do for her. She came in many times to talk and sent me lots of emails that were filled with mixed emotions. In the end, she wasn't completely satisfied with her results, even though she looked very good. Looking back, I realize that she wasn't good at explaining what she wanted, and she never really heard and connected with my explanations about her physique and specific skin qualities that would affect her surgical outcome. She heard only what she wanted to hear, and she couldn't let go of the images in her mind of what she wanted to look like versus what was possible. I delivered an excellent surgical result for her body, but I failed to manage her expectations, and I failed to recognize the red flags regarding her desires.

Good communication between you and your surgeon is necessary to arrive at realistic results. This means doing a lot of homework before going to your consultation so that you can be specific and describe in great detail what you don't like about your body now, what you want, and what you expect your surgical outcome to be. You should be able to honestly assess your reasons for wanting surgery, understand and assess the options your surgeon will tell you are right for you, and then, if needed, adjust your goals and expectations to meet reality.

If you went for a surgery consultation today, could you describe in detail what you don't like about your body and what you want? For example, someone wanting a breast procedure might ask herself the following questions to get to the details her surgeon needs:

- **What don't I like about my breasts?** (She might discuss breast size or cup size, shape, the nipple position, even the skin quality.)

- **What do I want?** (Hopefully she has photos of what she likes and wants and has done her research; these would help her communicate the desired size, shape, degree of fullness, and general look.)

- **Does it matter if people know I've had augmentation?** (This can be important, because some women don't care if they look augmented while others care a lot if people know they've had surgery.)

You can see the level of detail in these questions, and you can expect to talk with your surgeon in this kind of detail. Being as specific as possible helps your surgeon give you what you want.

After the first consultation, I ask patients to gather lots of photos of what they want to look like, and this is particularly important for breast augmentation procedures, especially before-and-after photos. I call this collection of photos a vision board, and done right, it can really save the surgeon from having to ask too many questions. You need to find the right photos. They shouldn't be images of a surgery result that you just happen to like, but rather images of women who are as close to you as possible in size, shape, body frame, and even skin quality. This is important because surgery results can be different from one woman to the next depending on all of those things. Ideally, when you bring the photos to your surgeon, you should be able to show a good comparison between yourself and the women in the photos. For example, "I'm as tall as that girl, her skin looks like it's the same quality as mine, and I feel like I'm looking at myself in her *before* picture. And, oh, by the way, I really love her after picture." You really need to compare like to like, so find before pictures that look like you.

IS THE PROCEDURE YOU WANT RIGHT FOR YOU?

Sometimes the particular procedure a patient wants might not be right for that individual, for any number of reasons. Some people just aren't good candidates for some procedures. For example, a patient wants fuller, rejuvenated breasts, but she isn't willing to have the scars that come with the procedure needed for the ideal result, which is a breast lift. This patient would be better off not having any surgery at all, because the procedure with less scars (just placing an implant without a lift) won't achieve the result she wants.

General health is the most important factor that overrides any other factor when considering who's a good candidate for any plastic-surgery procedure. Anyone who has many medical problems has a higher risk for complications from surgery. Some patients think they're perfectly healthy when in reality, they really aren't, and they don't understand the complications associated with surgery. I've turned patients away who aren't healthy enough to undergo an elective procedure, because the risk of a negative outcome increases. In these cases, life prevails over an elective procedure.

Here are some general health factors that make patients less-than-ideal candidates for surgery. Having these factors doesn't necessarily exclude a patient from having surgery, but the patient might require extra precautions. If you have any of these conditions, you must discuss them with your surgeon.

- Diabetes

- Hypertension

- Known bleeding or clotting disorder

- Cardiac disease

- Kidney disease

- Liver disease

- Asthma, chronic obstructive pulmonary disease, or other lung condition

- Obesity (High Body Mass Index)

- Smoking

- History of obstructive sleep apnea or excessive snoring

I've also turned patients away because what they want simply won't work for the bodies they have, and doing the procedure would likely result in something they'd regret later in life. For example, a patient wanted a breast augmentation, but she wanted to be much, much bigger than her small frame should carry. I looked her squarely in the face and said, "These implants are going to harm your body in the long term, and if you insist on doing this, I'm not the surgeon for you." I've talked with women who did what she wanted and now, in their sixties, they say they wish they'd never done it. Unfortunately, the women who surgeons turn away will often find a different surgeon who'll do the procedure for them despite the probable long-term impact. These women, too, will probably regret it later in life. I'm not saying that patients can't and shouldn't get large implants, but the implants do need to fit their body type.

To help you understand what makes someone a good or bad candidate for a specific procedure, let's look at the tummy tuck.

Patients might not be good candidates for a tummy tuck if they can answer "yes" to any of the following questions:

- **Do you intend to have more children?** The skin will just stretch and become saggy again, and you'll be right back to where you were.

- **Do you still need to lose a lot of weight?** You'll have saggy skin again once you lose more weight.

- **Are you already small but with just a little bit of loose skin?** A small amount of loose skin may not warrant making huge scars on the body to remove it; however, if that skin is just below the belly button, a mini–tummy tuck might work.

- **Do you need just a little bit of debulking of the subcutaneous tissue?** Liposuction may achieve your goal, and it's a lesser procedure.

Similarly, patients might not be good candidates for a breast procedure if they can answer "yes" to any of the following questions:

- **Are you not willing to have the scars that come with breast procedures?** All of these procedures produce scars—*all of them.*

- **Do you want a breast implant that's too large for your body?**

- **Have you had radiation treatment to a breast and want implants?** Radiation makes the skin tight and inflexible, and you can get painful contracture—internal scar tissue around the implant—because the tissue won't stretch.

- **Have you had radiation in the chest area, even if it wasn't directly to a breast?** An example is a patient who had a type of lymphoma that required radiation to the chest behind the sternum. In this case, the treatment likely irradiated the breast, too, and the patient might not be a great candidate for augmentation because of pain and contracture over time.

Women who've had radiation for breast cancer could still have reconstruction surgery, because they no longer have breast tissue. It's a completely different situation, and there are ways to augment breasts with their own tissue and implants.

For liposuction, patients might not be good candidates if they can answer "yes" to any of the following questions:

- **Are you too thin?** Some people who are quite thin actually come in and want liposuction, and I can't even find anything to take out.

- **Are you too large?** Some patients are so large that liposuction may not make any significant difference at all.

- **Do you have bad skin quality?** Older people with poor-quality collagen, for example, can still have liposuction, but the loose skin won't contract and tighten up on its own.

- **Do you have a disease like lymphedema?** Lymphedema is swelling in one or more extremities caused by impaired flow of the lymphatic system. People with this disease have large, thick legs—not from fat, but from a different process. Because it's not fat, liposuction won't work for them.

REALISTIC AND UNREALISTIC EXPECTATIONS

Unrealistic expectations about plastic-surgery results aren't automatically the end of the road. A good rapport, trust, and honest communication between the surgeon and patient might turn unrealistic expectations into realistic ones by getting to the root of the expectations.

Most patients can be quite clear about what they don't like about their bodies. Suppose someone says, "I hate these saddlebags on the outsides of my hips. Can we lipo those down?" The answer is "yes." But suppose someone who's very heavy wants liposuction because she thinks it's going to make her look like a supermodel. Well, that's just not going to happen, and that's what I have to tell her. This is a great example of how a procedure can be different depending on the patient—in this case, a very large person wanting liposuction versus someone who's lean but has a trouble area, like some fat on the outer hip or the love handle area. Liposuction for larger patients is a debulking procedure that reduces the volume so that clothes feel better and aren't as tight on her body. For the thinner patient with a problem area, the procedure will debulk, but it'll also contour and sculpt her and make her more curvy. So, I have to make that distinction to patients, because some larger patients think they'll be getting curves, and that's often not realistic.

Similarly, doing a tummy tuck on someone who still needs to lose eighty or one hundred pounds will remove extra skin and result in clothes that fit better. But doing a tummy tuck on a mom who's fairly lean and just has a lot of stretched-out skin with stretch marks on the lower part of her tummy will recontour the body, and she'll be more curvy and have better shape. The person who still needs to lose weight can't realistically expect her tummy tuck to make her more curvy and have better shape. That said, many people don't want or expect to be more curvy. They just want extra skin removed and for the surgeon to liposuction as much as possible, which makes them extremely happy. Everyone's desires and needs are different, and procedures aren't "one size fits all."

Anatomy is a big factor in what can or can't be done realistically. Every woman's body is asymmetric in some way, sometimes so subtly that she may not even see it herself. Almost everyone is imperfect to start. People with asymmetries who expect perfection are automatically set up for failure. The surgeon's job (and what I think is an important job) is to show them these asymmetries, thus setting them up for success. When I show patients their asymmetries, they can understand that maybe I can't fix them after all—but maybe I could enhance them, and they're prepared for that. I once told a woman that one breast might be a bit higher than the other one after surgery because of her body's asymmetry. Knowing about it beforehand, she accepted it, but if I hadn't told her, she could have been really unhappy with the result. Similarly, putting implants into someone with a congenital breast irregularity on one side could result in implants that don't look exactly alike anatomically. The skin might stretch and even out in time, but then again, it might not. This is common, and I sometimes tell such patients, "Don't expect twins— they're sisters."

I sometimes find things in my initial examination which tell me that what the patient wants isn't realistic, and I'll explain why what she is asking for won't work. But I can usually come up with an alternative plan that I think could achieve her goals.

Sometimes the "rules" can bend a bit for a patient who genuinely has realistic expectations.

I had a patient who looked me squarely in the face and said, "I'm not going to lose any more weight. If you can just take off this extra skin on the lower part of my tummy, I'm going to be really happy. And I'm not expecting you to make me super flat, and I don't expect to look like a model."

I was okay with that because her expectation was totally realistic. I knew that I could remove the extra skin, and she'd be a lot flatter than she was, but in no way would she look in the mirror and think she looked like a model. She knew that, and that was okay.

WILL I NEED ADDITIONAL SURGERY LATER IN LIFE?

Do procedures have a shelf life? Patients commonly ask me this question. Many factors are involved in sustaining surgery results, and an important factor is how well patients care for themselves afterward. (This is so important that I discuss it in more detail in part 3.)

What are some other factors? Age is important. When I see women in their twenties for breast augmentation, I tell them honestly, "You'll probably need one or two more operations in your lifetime. You need to be aware of that." She might have children at some point, and her breasts might change. She might not have children, but the quality of her skin and tissue will change with time, and she'll need a revision. She might want to be bigger or smaller, and therefore want another procedure.

Anatomy is also a factor, and no two patients are the same. I might know that a patient's breast lift will need revision in six months to a year simply because her anatomy limits how tight I can make the skin envelope. She would need the revision soon, because her skin quality is more lax than that of another patient with very good skin quality, and that patient might not need revision for years, if ever.

In breast implant cases, the implant itself can determine if the patient will need more surgeries. Implants have a shelf life, and no one can put a number on it. They're artificial devices that can fail, and any woman considering implants needs to understand that she'll probably have other implant-related operations on her breasts in her lifetime. I'm very clear with patients that implant surgery isn't a one-and-done deal, and it's the biggest discussion I have with patients about additional surgeries.

Pregnancy is another consideration. Suppose a woman in her mid-twenties doesn't want to have kids for ten years—but neither does she want to wait to have breast augmentation. I understand completely that she doesn't want to wait, but she might need a breast lift after having children. Some women do need it and some don't—it all depends on how her breasts react after being pregnant. Pregnancy especially affects tummy tucks. It's pointless to have a tummy tuck and then have children, because you just wreck the procedure and would end up needing another one. So, I usually do the procedure only on someone who either knows she doesn't want to have children or is done having children.

One simple factor affects liposuction: if you gain more weight, you're going to need more liposuction. You might not need as much in one area versus another, because the number of fat cells in the body is finite. When the fat cells are removed, they're gone forever and don't regrow. But the fat cells left behind can get bigger—that's how people can still regain weight after having liposuction. This clearly shows why it's important, postsurgery, to develop and maintain a new lifestyle that includes exercise, good nutrition, getting plenty of sleep, and stopping smoking. (This topic is so important that I discuss it in detail in chapter 14.)

CHAPTER 3

How Do I Talk with My
Family and Friends?

Are you feeling a bit hesitant to talk with your family and friends about your surgery? You're not alone, and it's normal. Deciding to have plastic surgery is deeply personal, so it's no surprise that you might find it hard to share your decision—and all the emotions that go with it—with friends and even close family. Maybe that's because family members sometimes don't easily accept a relative's decision to have plastic surgery. So, naturally, someone who wants surgery might fear their criticism or judgment and not know how to tell them. But it's important to open this line of communication with family, because if you can be honest with them, you can involve them in the process, and you'll want and need their support. If I hadn't asked my mom if I could have a rhinoplasty, I never would have known that she had one at my age and understood where I was coming from completely.

People hesitate to open up about their surgery for a lot of reasons. A woman might not want to tell her husband, because she fears he might dismiss what she wants and insist that he likes her just the way she is. She might also be afraid of what her kids will think and how they'll react. Family and friends often tell patients that they don't understand why having surgery is necessary or important. Some simply have negative opinions about it in general. All of this can cause patients to avoid talking about their upcoming surgery and thus avoid negative comments and difficult conversation. It's especially hard for men who want surgery—and more men are having plastic-surgery procedures today than ever before. Yet, there's still more stigma attached to men having surgery than women, and this is why women are more open to discussing it with others than men are—however, the Plastic Surgery Statistics Report by the American Society of Plastic Surgeons show one of the biggest upticks in male plastic surgery as of 2017.[2] Remember that you're doing this for yourself, and you deserve to feel the way you want to feel, so it really doesn't matter what everyone else thinks. Still, you do have to deal with family and friends.

On the plus side, telling others can bring you a sense of relief and take a load off your shoulders. If others know, you don't have to hide anything. It's not as if all the people you know are 100 percent happy with their own bodies, so it might be easier than you think for them to understand your desire to make some changes. After all, this is the twenty-first century, and people in general are more open about having plastic surgery, because society is more accepting. Plastic surgery isn't done in secret like it was decades ago, when patients told virtually no one and simply explained their time away as a "relaxing vacation, and boy, do I feel better!"

---

2   Josh Sabarra, "I Know Why More Men Are Getting Plastic Surgery – I was One of Them," Healthline, July 20, 2018, https://www.healthline.com/health-news/i-know-why-more-men-are-getting-plastic-surgery#4.

If you're concerned about telling family and friends, think about a few things before starting any discussions. Consider the following questions:

- Do you know how your family member (husband, wife, partner, parent, or child) feels about plastic surgery and people who want it?

- Does your family member have fears about your safety during plastic surgery, or fears about any surgery?

- Might a husband, wife, or partner be concerned that if you have surgery, your relationship might be in trouble because you'll be more beautiful or look younger?

- Might your family member think that spending money on plastic surgery is frivolous?

- Are you afraid that others will criticize or judge you?

- Are you concerned that family and friends might not understand your reasons for wanting surgery?

- Do you think they might simply believe you don't need surgery?

- Are you afraid that everyone will try to give you nonstop advice against having surgery?

- Are you afraid that people will shame you for being vain?

Considering these questions can help you plan whom to tell and how to answer negative reactions. It's important to think about and plan your conversations because having surgery can be stressful enough without adding more stress from family, who you hope will support you.

Tips for Preparing to Tell Family and Friends

Deciding whom to tell and how to tell them is your first step. Here are a few tips to help you through this process.

- Test the waters first. Casually find out peoples' attitudes toward plastic surgery well before you have your procedure. This will help you decide who to tell and who to skip.

- Think about a good environment for your talk. You might not want to do it in public, so depending on who you plan to tell, dinner at home or a walk in the park could be good alternatives.

- Tell the "easy" ones first. Figure out who is likely to be the most supportive, and talk with those people first. It'll help break the ice for you and give you more confidence to tell others.

- Get your ducks in a row. In other words, have your reasons ready, and plan how you might bring someone around to understand your desire for surgery.

- Be honest, straightforward, and matter-of-fact. Tell them why you want to have surgery and how you think doing so will make you feel about yourself and boost your self-confidence.

TELLING THE KIDS

Should you tell your children about your plastic surgery? That's entirely up to you. You know your kids better than anyone else does, so you probably have a feel for how they might react. Kids today are a lot more sophisticated about things like plastic surgery thanks to reality TV and the Internet, so telling them might not be as big a deal as you think. They might even think you're really cool for doing something like this. If you don't already know how much exposure your kids have to the subject, find out. It could make the whole discussion a lot easier.

Some people decide that their kids just won't understand, so they plan their surgery for when the kids are at summer camp, or they send them to relatives for a nice, long vacation. Maybe this isn't such a bad idea if the kids are young and aren't mature enough understand. Other people just sit down and talk with their kids about it the same way they'd talk with their adult family and friends. This could be the best approach with older kids who might know a lot about it.

If you decide to tell your kids, the following suggestions can make the conversation easier:

- Keep it simple. Explain things without big words or complex ideas.

- Avoid talking about highly technical things about surgery, and downplay the pain aspect. You don't want to confuse or upset them.

- Tell them you're doing it to feel good, and that it's okay to do that.

Tips for Preparing to Tell Family and Friends (continued)

- Don't tell the ones that you think just won't get it. Honestly, you don't have to tell everyone, and if telling someone will cause more stress and anxiety than it's worth, then don't tell them.

- Be prepared for surprises. Someone will always surprise you, and not always the way you hope. You might think someone will be supportive, but what if it doesn't turn out that way? Think about how you'll react to such surprises.

- Develop a thick skin. Be ready to react gracefully to any negative reactions from those you tell.

You might also consider telling as few people as possible. Nothing says you have to tell all of your family or everyone you know. In fact, depending on your situation, maybe saying less to fewer people would work out best for you.

- Let them know that they're perfect just the way they are. Kids might think that if you're "fixing" yourself, maybe there's something "wrong" with them, too. Make sure they understand that this is something you're doing because you want to—you don't *need to do it*—*and they shouldn't think there's anything wrong with them.*

IT'S ABOUT YOU

Probably the most important thing for any of your family and friends to know is that your decision to have surgery isn't about any of them—not your spouse, parents, friends, kids, or anyone else. This is about you wanting to feel better about yourself, look better in your clothes (or while being intimate), and look as good as you feel. You're doing it for yourself and no one else, and sometimes, that's really all any of them needs to hear.

CHAPTER 4

Choosing the Right Plastic Surgeon for You

I want to say this right up front: There is no board-certification in *cosmetic* surgery. Period. The only board-certification that's relevant to cosmetic procedures and that means anything when you're looking for the right surgeon is the American Board of Plastic Surgery (ABPS). This board certifies plastic surgeons who are cosmetic and reconstructive surgeons. All plastic surgeons are cosmetic and reconstructive surgeons, but not all surgeons who call themselves cosmetic surgeons are plastic and reconstructive surgeons. Anyone who has a medical degree can use the title of cosmetic surgeon, but only someone who has undergone rigorous training, residencies, and oral and written exams in plastic and reconstructive surgery can become a board-certified plastic surgeon.

Choosing the surgeon who'll perform your procedures is the most important factor you can control that leads to successful outcomes.

Board-certification is the key to finding a skilled, knowledgeable, competent, and safe surgeon, and the only board that matters is the ABPS. Before you do anything else, visit the ABPS website to read an article on why you should choose an ABPS-certified plastic surgeon.[3]

The ABPS tests surgeons first with a written exam of more than four hundred questions. Only physicians who pass that exam will move on to a rigorous, two-day oral examination on cases they've done and on unknown cases, and the surgeons' peers scrutinize them besides. Although none of this means that all board-certified surgeons are good surgeons, board-certified surgeons have had training to be safe at what they do. Their peers have determined that they have the skill set and knowledge to be safe surgeons and perform all the cosmetic and reconstructive procedures in the field of plastic surgery. Candidates for board certification sit in front of surgeons who've been practicing in the field for a very long time, and these surgeons ask questions to determine if the candidates handled the scenarios safely.

When you find one or more board-certified surgeons to consider, you still have more work to do. You still need to research their reputations. Just because they passed the test and the oral exams doesn't mean that they're ethical. It doesn't mean that they use best practices or follow the Hippocratic Oath. So, it's still up to you to figure out if a physician uses best practices, has good results and treats patients with respect, has a good bedside manner, stands behind his or her work, and has helpful, respectful staff. Look at online reviews, check out the before-and-after photos on the surgeon's website, and ask the surgeon if you can talk with patients about their experiences. Board-certification doesn't automatically mean a surgeon is awesome and always gets amazing results. You still need to dig a little deeper.

---

3   "Why Choose an ABCS Surgeon?" American Board of Cosmetic Surgery, https://www.americanboardcosmeticsurgery.org/patient-resources/choose-abcs-surgeon.

I think you should pay close attention to your comfort level with a surgeon and the staff, kind of go with your gut feelings. People get intuitive feelings from being with someone. If you feel as though the surgeon or his staff is rushing you, don't ignore that feeling. Patients have told me that some physicians will rush them straight to the exam if the patient doesn't ask any immediate questions. The first interaction goes something like this: "Hey, nice to meet you. Did you have any more questions about the tummy tuck? Well, great. Let's just take a quick look, and we'll get you a quote, and I'll see you for pre-op if you want to sign up. Okay, bye." This isn't great bedside manner, and if you do meet a physician like this, you should definitely say goodbye.

Checklist for Finding the Right Plastic Surgeon for You

- Is the surgeon board-certified by the American Board of Plastic Surgery? This is the most important item.
- Is the surgeon a member of the American Society of Plastic Surgery?
- Is the surgeon a member of the American Society of Aesthetic Plastic surgery?
- Does the surgeon have experience in the procedures you want?
- Have you seen the surgeon's work, and do you like what you see?
- Do you feel comfortable with the surgeon—comfortable enough to discuss all the details of your medical history?
- Do you feel like you can trust the surgeon to do the right things for you?
- Do you feel that this surgeon considers safety to be a high priority?
- Do you like the surgeon's staff and feel comfortable with them?

Checklist for Finding the Right Plastic Surgeon for You (continued)

- Does the surgeon and the staff treat you courteously and behave professionally?

- Do you like what you see in the surgeon's office and other facilities?

- Does the surgeon understand what you want and what you expect?

- Do the surgeon and the staff listen to you and answer your concerns?

- Does the surgeon spend time with you, or do you feel rushed?

- Is the surgeon available to answer the questions you're almost certain to have after your consultation? Can you contact the surgeon by phone or email with your questions?

- Does the staff make you feel welcome?

- Does the staff explain the financial aspects of your surgery in detail? Do they answer all of your questions about finances?

You should never feel hurried, and you should feel trust in the office environment. You should feel as if the physician and staff are educating you and not rushing you into anything. When you leave the office, you should feel you've had a positive—even awesome—experience and ask yourself the following questions:

- Do I feel less nervous than I was when I arrived?

- Did I get the education I need?

- Do I understand exactly what's involved and expected of me financially?

- Do I know exactly what's going to happen to me if I have a complication postoperatively, and what that means for me financially?

If you can answer only "no" to those questions, keep looking because you haven't yet found the right surgeon for you.

RED FLAGS

Be on the lookout for red flags that tell you a surgeon might not be the right one for you. The following should cause concern about any physician you're considering:

- Isn't board-certified by the American Board of Plastic Surgery

- Has bad reviews online

- Has no reviews online

- Has bad photos online or on their website

- Has no photos—anywhere

- Has a dismissive attitude

- Is in a hurry and won't spend time with you in thoughtful discussion

- Doesn't actually do an exam

- Trash talks other surgeons

- Doesn't have hospital privileges

- Doesn't use accredited surgical facilities

- Doesn't listen to you, but just talks and spouts knowledge

- Tries to push procedures on you that you aren't interested in having

- Won't show you before-and-after photos

- Is unwilling to let you talk with a patient who's happy with the procedure that you want

- Isn't available to answer questions after your consultation

MORE RESOURCES

The surgery you're considering can be life changing and is a big financial investment, so you should spare nothing in doing the most extensive research you can beforehand, especially about the surgeon you choose. You need to be knowledgeable when you go to your consultation. The websites of the following professional organizations have a lot of important information that you can use:

- American Board of Medical Specialties: http://www.abms.org

- American Board of Plastic Surgery: https://www.abplasticsurgery.org

- American Society of Plastic Surgery: https://www.plasticsurgery.org

- American Society of Aesthetic Plastic Surgery: https://www.surgery.org

BAD PLASTIC SURGERY—WHAT COULD GO WRONG?

Choosing the right surgeon is crucial to avoiding bad plastic surgery. We've all heard stories and read the screaming headlines about things that go wrong because a physician performed complicated plastic surgery procedures without the rigorous training and testing that board-certification requires. I've even seen dentists advertising that they do breast augmentation! Seriously, I've seen it, and I've corrected their bad results. Frankly, I don't understand how someone could even consider going to a dentist thinking, "I want you to do my breast augmentation," but it happens, and it's probably not a good idea. I never judge someone who comes to me to repair a bad result from someone like that, but I have to be honest that fixing it usually ends up costing as much as three times what the patient thought an augmentation would cost.

Unfortunately, bad plastic surgery can make people think that all plastic surgery is dangerous, and that's simply not true. Plastic surgery performed by people who aren't trained properly and aren't board-certified—that's what's dangerous.

As I write this, I've recently performed revisions on a patient who had a dentist do her breast augmentation ten years ago, and it was never right from the beginning. I've also had patients come to me who'd originally gone to Mexico for the procedure, had to go back for a revision, then went back again five years later to have yet another revision—and it still didn't look right. You can avoid this if you're careful and make sure to choose a well-trained, board-certified surgeon to ensure competency and safety. If you need open-heart surgery, will you choose the least-expensive surgeon to operate on your heart, or will you choose the most talented and experienced surgeon with the credentials and reputation to back it up? Choosing your plastic surgeon is the same. Don't be cheap and take risks with your body, because your body is the only one you have!

MAKING THE MOST OF YOUR PLASTIC-SURGERY CONSULTATION

It's exciting to prepare for and have your surgery consultation. What should you expect from it? You'll have an intellectual conversation with your surgeon about your goals and whether they're accomplishable or if they're somewhere in between what you want and what's realistic. The goal of the consultation is for you and the surgeon to arrive at what you both agree would be your perfect outcome. The surgeon will describe what the procedure entails and answer all of your questions about what you'll experience from start to finish. You should leave your consultation feeling completely educated about the procedure, the risks, and the expected outcomes. You should leave with few, if any, unanswered questions and know how the whole experience will go from pre-op to surgery, to recovery, and afterward.

You can expect most surgeons to charge a consultation fee. It's necessary because the consultation takes time; it's our work, and most people don't work for nothing. You wouldn't believe how many consultation appointments turn into no-shows, and that's wasted time that a physician could use to see other patients. Some offices ask for credit card information and will charge a fee if you don't show up. Now, this is where all the research you do on finding the right surgeon starts to work for you. Make a list of the top five surgeons you're willing to see—the ones your research shows have the reputation, results, and expertise you want—and have a budget for consultations with those surgeons. Be comfortable spending $400–$500 worth of consultation fees to get the right surgeon—it's that important. In many cases, the surgeon will credit your fee toward your procedure if you choose that surgeon.

BEFORE THE CONSULTATION

To prepare for the consultation, you should have a sense of what you want and what you think you want to look like. Be prepared to explain in good detail, as best you can, what you don't like about your body and what you think the procedure or procedures can accomplish. Bring anything with you that can help the surgeon understand what you want. I ask patients to look at a lot of before-and-after pictures to find people with similar physiques and body types to their own, who are in their approximate age group, and if possible, have similar life circumstances. This is very important. Those photos are the vision board I described in chapter 2, and it can really benefit both you and your surgeon.

You might also bring an extra pair of ears—a friend or a spouse—because it can be comforting if you're a bit nervous. The physician and staff will be giving you a lot of information, and it's good to have someone else listening in case you don't hear everything, or if you hear something different from what the surgeon said. It's often good to bring along a friend who's had a procedure, because someone who has been through it can help you ask the right questions.

Your first encounter with a surgeon's office will be on the phone when you call to make the appointment. Don't expect to receive detailed medical information or even financial details on the phone—you'll have to wait until you come in for your appointment. The person answering the phone can't give you information that requires the physician's expertise, and they can't quote specific procedure costs, because no one can possibly know exactly what you need until the physician sees you. Every patient is different, and procedures vary.

THE CONSULTATION

Your consultation usually involves a lot of people, from the front-office staff to patient coordinators, medical assistants, and financial people. You might fill out some medical forms when you first check in if you didn't or couldn't get them beforehand and fill them out at home. Generally, your first contact will be with medical assistants who take your detailed medical history. At some point, you'll meet with the financial person to discuss finances.

Some offices have you meet with the medical assistant or coordinator alone, before seeing the physician. These people are knowledgeable and can answer consultation questions before you see the physician for the exam. We do this in my office sometimes, and I tell patients that they're choosing my office as much as they're choosing me. The people who work for me interact with patients the same way that I would. I spend a lot of time developing my staff so patients feel comfortable with them. This brings up a point: in general, if any patients find that they like the doctor they chose but don't like the staff, that's a problem. I've had patients tell me that they chose me over another surgeon simply because they didn't like the other surgeon's staff.

You get into the fine details of the procedure you want when you meet with the surgeon. The physician will ask you a lot of questions

Types of Questions a Surgeon Might Ask

Surgeons will ask you highly detailed questions to understand what you want and what you expect. For a breast augmentation, for example, a surgeon might ask questions like these:

- How big do you want to be? What's too big? What's too small?

- Are you afraid to be too large or too small?

- Are you being realistic or unrealistic about the size of the implant for your body?

- Are you looking for a breast that looks teardrop-shaped or full and round?

- Do you desire saline or silicone?

- Do you care if you look "augmented?"

that are specific to your issues and your procedure, and you should be prepared to tell the surgeon in detail what you don't like about your body, what you expect from the surgery, and what your reasons are for doing it. The physician will try to make sure that your expectations are reasonable and that you understand what's possible and what isn't. Other details the surgeon will cover include where you'll have the procedure, anesthesia, recovery, and what to expect in the long term after surgery. Understanding all of these factors is important to you making an informed decision.

If you go into the consultation expecting the surgeon to tell you what you need, you might not be ready for a consultation. A good surgeon will try to coax the information out of you through detailed, thorough questioning. If you're a bit vague with details, your vision board photos can help a lot.

AFTER THE CONSULTATIONS

Now that you've seen several plastic surgeons and met many office staff members, what do you do? How do you choose? Start by making a list of all the doctors, using your first impressions to rank them. (Often your first instincts are correct.) Next, reorganize your list based on the staff you met. Now you can see which physician *and* staff you liked. Number one on your list is usually the right surgeon for you, but something might also draw you to another particular office. If that happens, make a list of the pros and cons of visiting each office to help narrow your choice further. It could even further validate your first choice.

Once you've chosen your surgeon and staff, your next step is to schedule your surgery. You're so excited that you want to do the procedure tomorrow because you've probably been waiting years for this! But like everything else about this process, picking your surgery date takes planning, because you have to get your schedule and your surgeon's schedule to agree. Think about dates that work for you and your family, and be flexible if possible. Surgeons tend to operate on specific days and not five days a week, so your first two choices might not be available if you choose a busy surgeon. It's best to find several dates that work for you, then call to schedule the surgery. Most surgeons require a deposit to hold your place on the surgery schedule. It could be several hundred dollars (I charge $500), and this deposit is applied to your total cost. Many offices won't refund this deposit if you cancel your surgery because the surgeon pays up-front costs to reserve the facility and the anesthesia staff. But if you simply reschedule your surgery, the surgeon would likely apply the fee toward your total cost. I discuss financial matters in more detail in the next chapter.

CHAPTER 5

Finances — How Can I Afford Surgery?

I believe everyone should have the plastic-surgery procedures they want if they're good candidates for it, but I think they should also be smart about it, financially. You're making a real investment in yourself when you decide to have surgery, and it's easy to get overextended. It's important to consider how you're going to finance what you want.

I'm a surgeon, not a financial advisor. But from what I've seen with patients through the years, I advise you to give a lot of thought to how you're going to finance your surgery without putting undue financial pressure on yourself. In other words, you probably shouldn't mortgage your house to have surgery. Remember, these are elective procedures, not emergencies. I realize that patients are excited to make these changes, but I think they need to ask themselves: "Is this right for me right now in my life? Can I afford it?" It's just about being responsible and not getting financially strapped. Remembering this can give you perspective when you think about how to finance your procedure.

To help you understand what you're paying for, I'll explain what's included in the cost of your surgery.

THE BUSINESS SIDE OF PLASTIC SURGERY

Surgeons have to pay several fees up front, so most require full payment two weeks before your surgery. There are three basic fees: for the anesthesiologist, the facility, and the surgeon. These basic fees could increase, too, if your procedure takes longer than expected. You'd spend more time in the facility, and the surgeon would use the anesthesiologist's services for longer than planned. If that happens, you'd have to cover those additional fees. Add-on fees are another part of the cost, and they vary depending on the procedure. For example, in implant surgery, the cost of the implants is an add-on. If the procedure needs a laser, the surgeon pays a rental fee. Compression garments and special medications also add to the cost, so you see how add-ons can add up. Generally, the physician pays for many or all of these costs up front.

Sometimes the hospital increases its anesthesia or facility fees, which means the patient's price increases. I try to avoid pricing surprises. I give patients a quote that's good for three months, but if any of those basic fees increases during that time, I pass the increase along to the patient. Most surgeons do business this way, because we typically see those fees raised at least yearly, sometimes twice a year. Your surgeon might own his or her own surgery center and can absorb some of those charges, but most surgeons use outpatient surgery centers that charge fees.

The possibility of needing unforeseen touch-ups can also add to costs. For example, a scar might need revision, or a patient decides she wants to exchange her implants for larger ones. Anything that requires going back into the operating room is going to incur all those fees again, and covering them will be the patient's responsibility. (If there's something I can do in the office instead of a surgery facility—such as reducing the visibility of breast augmentation scars, which don't require any sedation or general anesthesia—I usually don't charge my patients if it's within reason, and it is 99 percent of the time.)

Two other situations are worth detailed discussion because they can also add to your procedure's costs.

REVISION SURGERY

Sometimes a patient isn't happy with the surgery results, but unless there's negligence involved, it's usually not the surgeon's fault. So what does this have to do with finances? Simply put, the surgeon will charge you for revision surgery that requires going back to the operating room. You might need to consider this when figuring out your surgery budget, depending on your procedure and the possibility of needing revisions. You likely won't need to concern yourself with this if you've chosen someone with an excellent reputation and who delivers excellent results, but in rare cases, even the best surgeons can have unhappy patients.

Asymmetry that can result from a liposuction procedure is an example—although the surgeon might consider any asymmetry from liposuction to be normal, the patient might not like it and would want it fixed. Another example involves implants that aren't the same size, because the breasts were naturally asymmetrical before surgery. In both examples, the surgeon would discuss these procedures' asymmetry risks in detail before the surgery, and the patient would sign an informed consent acknowledging that she understands and accepts these risks. So, it's pretty clear from the start that asymmetries like this happen; everyone knows they happen; and if they do, it takes another surgery to fix it—incurring another charge for the revision.

STAGED PROCEDURES

Some procedures need more than one surgery for safety reasons. You'll find out in your consultation if your procedure might need this staging. (I'm mentioning this in the finances section, because you'll have to pay those up-front fees each time you have an operation.)

Which procedures might require staging? It depends on you, the patient, and what risks your procedure might pose for you. Let's say a patient comes in for an arm lift. This patient is fairly heavy and has rather large arms, or maybe just has a lot of fatty tissue in her arms. I might decide to stage the procedure. I'd do an aggressive liposuction procedure first to debulk, but I couldn't cut the excess skin out at that time, because liposuction can create swelling making it difficult to take enough skin out safely. This is because, sometimes larger patients need to be debulked first with liposuction, then allow swelling and tissues to recover. I'd plan a second procedure to remove the skin in a couple of months when it's safer to do so and swelling has resolved, and this would get the best result. Other procedures that could require staging are a combined breast augmentation and lift, and a circumferential body lift performed after massive weight-loss surgery (This entails a traditional tummy tuck in front but continuing the incision around the backside to lift the outer thighs and butt).

Sometimes a patient wants multiple procedures and expects to have them all done at the same time. Breasts, arms, thighs, tummy—

she wants to do it all and has the money to do it. But is it safe to do all of that at once? No. All that surgery at one time is just too much, and there's a point where it becomes unsafe to keep a patient on the table that long because complication rates go up drastically. Besides, I'd be taking both the arms and legs out of commission at the same time, and the patient wouldn't be able to move, walk, or pick anything up. So, this is another example of needing multiple, separate surgeries, and they all come with their respective fees.

HOW TO PAY FOR YOUR SURGERY

CASH

You can pay for part of your procedure in cash. My office doesn't accept more than $8,000 in cash, but we'll take a personal check or cashier's check for the balance. Some of my patients felt that they didn't need to have the surgery right now, and they were willing to wait for what they wanted until they'd saved the money to pay for it without going deeply into debt. I liked that attitude in them. To me, it showed how much they cared about themselves, not only because they were going to give themselves the surgery they wanted, but also because they planned for it financially. It's something to consider.

CREDIT

You might decide to use credit cards, and that's okay. You can also apply for credit through companies like CareCredit or Alphaeon Credit, which are like medical credit cards. You can research other, similar medical-credit companies.

PHYSICIAN PAYMENT PLANS

Some physicians will set up a payment plan, and you just pay the doctor monthly until you pay it off, but usually you need to do that before they'll even schedule your procedure. It's like lay-away surgery, and it's a great idea because you pay for it slowly so that you don't need to mortgage the house. Plus, if you've paid the practice, the money's not sitting around where you'll spend it.

Again, surgery is expensive. But if you plan appropriately and budget correctly, you can have your cake and eat it, too—you should just be diligent and smart about how you do it. Even if you have to put off your procedure until you've saved enough money, you'll be glad you planned for it and didn't go deeply into debt.

PART 2

What You Need to Know About Popular Procedures

Now that you've decided to have surgery, I'll give you basic information about some of the most popular plastic-surgery procedures so that you'll understand the overall principles. Your physician will describe the procedures that interest you in much more detail during your consultation. I'm just giving you an overall view of the surgery experience, the types of incisions you should expect, healing times, and other general information.

Each procedure has specific pre and postsurgery instructions, but some instructions generally apply to all of the procedures in the next several chapters. These include the following:

Surgery preparation: Discuss your medical history and medications with your surgeon. If you use nicotine products, you'll need to stop for four weeks before and after surgery.

Restrictions after surgery: Generally, you can shower in one to two days after surgery, but no baths, hot tubs, or swimming pools for three weeks minimum.

Playing sports after surgery: Physically active patients who play sports can be passionate about their lives and the sports they play, and usually they're anxious to get back to competing again as soon as possible after surgery. Everyone wants a speedy recovery, but those who want to return to playing sports have some extra considerations. Because every procedure is different, it often depends on the procedure and how much the specific sport you play will affect the treated area. For example, going back to playing a physically demanding sport such as soccer after breast-enhancement surgery might require some time and patience. You want to make sure that you're healing correctly and on pace with what your surgeon expects, but you also want to make sure that enough recovery time has passed so you don't feel any unnecessary pain. Your surgeon will advise you every step of the way and have a major role in your ability to get back to playing your sport again quickly. Be sure to tell your surgeon about your favorite sport in your early consultation—long before you have your surgery—so you're fully aware of the expectations and have a realistic time frame in mind. Like me, your surgeon's goal for patients is a complete healing process, and even though you might be anxious to get back into the swing of things sooner rather than later, it's important for your body to heal 100 percent.

Travel after surgery: Most patients are eager to get back to their normal lifestyles as quickly and as safely as possible after any surgery. Many of my patients look forward to getting back to their favorite activities after surgery, like traveling, but you can't travel right away.

You should not drive until your surgeon clears you. Generally, this is when you are off of mind-altering medications, and are pain-free enough to maneuver a car in an emergency. You should avoid air travel, long-distance car trips, train rides, and the like until after your first postoperative visit, which is usually five to seven days after surgery. If your surgeon identified you as a high-risk patient for blood clots, you shouldn't travel at all after surgery until your physician says you can.

Problems after surgery: If you have any concerns at all after your procedure, call your surgeon.

The next chapters cover basic information about breast, body, and gluteal procedures, along with information about a group of procedures known as the Mommy Makeover, and procedures to tighten and tone patients who've had weight-loss surgery for obesity.

CHAPTER 6

Breast Procedures

Breast-enhancement procedures are probably the most popular surgeries for women. Regardless of age or how many children they've had, I see them achieve their realistic goals and have the breasts they've always wanted. Women who've had children and those who haven't but were born with small breasts or no breasts; women with saggy, hanging breasts; young women in their late twenties with the tissue quality of a seventy-year-old woman—they all come in wanting enhancement for many reasons. For example, some don't feel feminine because they were born with boyish-looking chests and they can't wear bras or bathing suits. They're so excited to have enhancement surgery, even if just adds a little volume. This surgery changes their lives and makes them feel so much better about themselves.

Sometimes men who have large breasts (gynecomastia) want breast reduction. They can be young, fit, and muscular, but if they take their shirts off, they look great except for their extra breast tissue. These guys can be so self-conscious about wearing tight t-shirts or bathing trunks, but it might take only a little liposuction to remove that tissue, and it's life-changing.

Interestingly, although breast-enhancement procedures are the most popular, breast-reduction surgery has the highest satisfaction rate of any procedure. Those patients are the happiest of all who undergo breast surgery, because the change is like night and day for them.

BREAST AUGMENTATION

Breast augmentation enhances the size and shape of a woman's breast. The surgeon uses various techniques to place the implant where it'll create a youthful contour to the existing breast tissue.

Initial consultation: You and your surgeon will determine the size and type of implants that are best for you and discuss the various surgical techniques best suited for you, based on the quality of your breast tissue and skin tone. If you have sagging breasts, the surgeon might suggest having a breast lift at the same time, which means additional scars related to the lift.

You won't always have to choose the exact implant you want immediately, but rather the consultation is a time for you to give the surgeon a general idea of the volume you want in an implant. You can go home and look at before-and-after photos of women who have the same breast type as you do to find some that you like, and then send them to the doctor before the preoperative visit. During this visit, you'll both hone in on a realistic outcome using the photos you sent. In my practice, I use silicone sizers to try different sizes of implants during the surgery to see what looks best for the patient's size and frame and for what they hope to achieve. (Not all surgeons do this.) Essentially, I end up picking the right size for the patient at that time, and the size is usually within a range that the patient and I discussed and agreed on before the surgery. Sometimes I have to decide to go outside of those ranges while the patient is on the table in order to achieve a look similar to their wish photos.

Surgery: Breast-augmentation surgery usually takes one hour to complete, plus another sixty to ninety minutes if combined with a breast-lift procedure. The surgeon places the implants through incisions in the armpit, the crease below the breast fold, or around the edge of the areola (the dark skin surrounding the nipple) and places them in a pocket created directly behind the breast tissue or underneath the pectoral muscle on the chest wall. Surgeons can perform breast augmentations in an outpatient setting or in the office under twilight or general anesthesia. For safety, I perform all augmentations under general anesthesia, and I'm also most comfortable performing them that way. I also use the Keller funnel,[4] a patented device that allows a no-touch technique to introduce the implant into the pocket, thus reducing contamination of the implant.

After breast augmentation surgery: Swelling and bruising are normal signs of healing. Swelling peaks at about forty-eight hours after surgery, then rapidly decreases, and 50 percent of swelling is gone by the end of the first few weeks. By six to eight weeks, most swelling has diminished, and by six months, almost all swelling is gone. Any remaining swelling is nearly imperceptible. You usually spend the first day after surgery lying in bed or sitting in a chair and should start walking around your house the day of surgery. You'll wear a surgical or sports bra for at least four to six weeks, and shouldn't do any vigorous activities or heavy lifting (more than twenty pounds)

---

4   "Keller Funnel," https://www.kellerfunnel.com.

until six weeks after surgery. These guidelines are general, and your surgeon will give you more specific instructions at your consultation.

BEFORE   **AFTER**

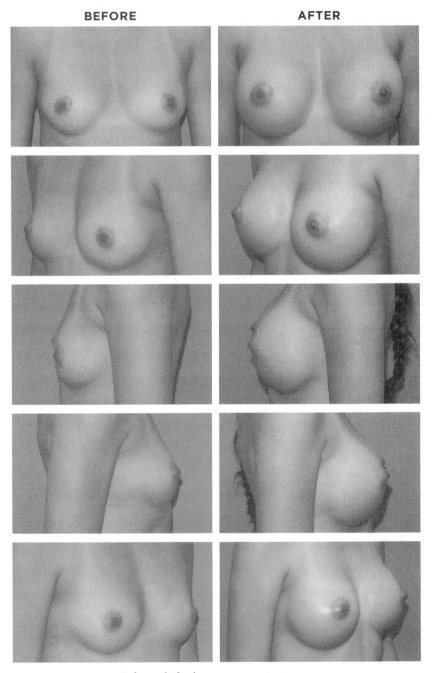

Before and after breast augmentation surgery.

Mammograms: All patients over the age of forty are required to have a mammogram within one year of surgery. You can continue your routine screening mammograms if you're age forty or older; if you're under forty and having annual mammograms because of a high-risk scenario, continue your screenings. In either case, always consult your women's-health practitioner for advice on mammograms. Be sure to have your screening at a radiology center with technicians experienced in the special techniques needed to obtain reliable images of the breast tissue.

SILICONE VERSUS SALINE IMPLANTS

Your surgeon will help you decide which implants are best for you, and this might be a function of your physiology, how much breast tissue you have, and the thickness or thinness of your skin. I think silicone is the better choice for patients with thin skin and thinner breast tissue because it feels softer, whereas saline tends to feel much firmer. Also, implants can have natural folds or ripples of the shell that are more palpable if there's not enough tissue covering them, so silicone is a better choice for thin-skinned patients, because it ripples less compared with saline. Both saline and silicone are good choices for patients with good-quality tissue, but ultimately, the physical exam and your personal preference determines which ones to use.

What are the major differences between the two? Generally, saline is firmer than silicone, and some patients don't like that. Silicone is soft, and therefore silicone implants feel softer. The upside to saline is that a ruptured implant releases only salt water and simply deflates—and you would know if this has happened right away. If silicone ruptures, though, it won't leak immediately because these gels are more cohesive. A patient who has a microperforation might not know it for years, or will notice slowly with time that the breast looks and feels different. However, there is no scientific data to date suggesting that silicone travels throughout the bloodstream and causes problems.

CORRECTING BREAST ASYMMETRY

I discussed in part 1 how nearly all women's breasts are asymmetric. Normal breast asymmetry will carry over to the result of enhancement surgery. But some women are born with highly asymmetric breasts—one might look perfectly normal, but the other is droopy and lacks volume, for example. Surgery can correct this and make them look much more alike. In the example case, one breast needs an implant and a lift to obtain as much symmetry as possible. I see these cases all the time and fix them.

IMPLANT REMOVAL

Some patients come into my office with breast implants that were placed by other surgeons or myself. There are many reasons why a patient may want to remove their implants. Some patients simply do not want them any longer. They are not as important as maybe they once were to them. For instance, say a seventy-year-old woman who has developed hard contractures, tightening of the capsules and of her implants comes to see me. Rather than having another surgery later in life, she may decide to remove the capsules and implants and not replace them. Oftentimes a patient will have a breast lift if needed at the same time. Other patients have had so many complications and attempted corrective procedures that have failed and decide to remove their implants all together.

There is one more reason that patients may request implant removal. That is the belief that implants are making them sick. This is not something that has been identified scientifically as a disease or problem. That is not to say that these women are wrong. There are many women who feel that, after placement of their breast implants, they began to notice medical problems like depression, thyroid problems, fatigue, malaise, and joint pain. This is not new to us as Dow Corning, the original breast implant company, was sued for this claim. The FDA found that these claims were not true, but they eventually went bankrupt anyway.

I believe Breast Implant Illness (or BII) is something that many surgeons shun women out of the office for and they are made to feel like they are crazy. I do not share that sentiment. As a scientist and a doctor, I would be crazy to tell a patient that it is impossible that their implants are making them feel sick. While we have no test to date that can prove implants make patients sick, and we do not have a test that can tell us who is susceptible, I do believe there could be a subset of patients who—for whatever reason—are prone to a chronic autoimmune or inflammatory response that makes them sick. So I will remove them freely for patients who have literally exhausted all other medical explanation for the way they feel to see if it makes them better. I want to be clear that while there are many women who say implants are making them feel sick, there are many, many more who have had implants for a long time and are just fine. I would never place breast implants if I felt that they were harming patients. So I do think they are safe and I will continue to use them for cosmetic and reconstructive purposes.

BEFORE **AFTER**

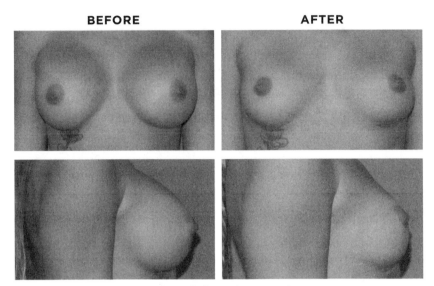

Before and after implant removal.

BREAST LIFT

A breast lift can rejuvenate breasts to appear more youthful and projecting. However, a lift won't change the size significantly or fill out the upper part of the breasts. This procedure will correct droopy breasts (breast ptosis), a condition seen mostly in patients who have lost a substantial amount of weight, and in childbearing women. It can be exaggerated in women who have breastfed their children. Sagging breasts are just part of growing older—the ligaments that support the breast on the chest wall stretch out with age, and the skin will, too. A lift combined with a breast augmentation can improve the breasts' volume and shape.

Initial consultation: You and your surgeon will discuss the results you want, which is important to choosing which technique to use. Generally, the larger and droopier the breast, the more skin the surgeon has to remove. Be sure to tell your surgeon if you plan to have children later, because pregnancy can affect the shape and size of your breasts. Having a lift before having kids could affect your surgery results.

Surgery: The surgery usually takes one to two hours to complete, plus another sixty to ninety minutes if performed with a breast augmentation. The degree of droopiness determines the type of incisions your surgeon will make. If they're not too droopy, an incision around the areola (the dark skin around the nipple) is all that's needed (Peri-areolar Lift). Moderately droopy breasts need that incision plus a vertical incision down the center of the breast (Lollipop Lift). Very droopy breasts need those two incisions and often need another horizontal incision along the lower breast crease (Anchor Lift).

After breast lift surgery: Normal swelling peaks at about forty-eight hours, quickly decreases to about 50 percent after the first few weeks, decreases even more in six to eight weeks, and is nearly gone by six months after surgery.

BEFORE	AFTER

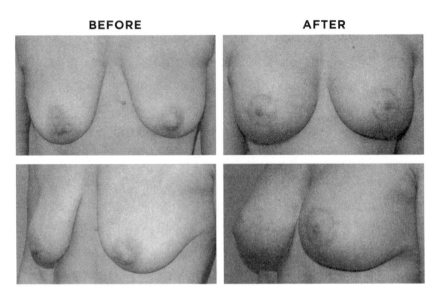

Before and after breast lift surgery.

BREAST REDUCTION

Breast reduction surgery reduces breast size and returns the breast to a more youthful, projecting shape, similar to a lift. Many women with large, heavy breasts have neck pain, back pain, and difficulty exercising. Reduction surgery can help improve these symptoms, though there's no guarantee you'll have symptom relief.

Initial consultation: Tell your surgeon if you plan to have children after the surgery and about any family or personal history of breast cancer. You'll discuss which surgical technique is most appropriate for you based on the size and shape of your breasts.

INSURANCE COVERAGE FOR REDUCTION SURGERY

Your physician may talk with you about insurance coverage for reduction surgery, but if not, be sure to bring it up. Health insurance might cover the cost. Insurance companies are finicky, and if you are a patient who really needs a breast lift, not a reduction, they will deny your case. Insurance companies individually determine who has a medically necessary case and who does not. The criteria by which they make that decision is not something your surgeon can control.

In the first case, the patient might not have enough breast tissue for reduction surgery and should have a breast lift instead. Many women I see in my practice think they need a reduction, but when I examine them, I might find that they don't have enough breast tissue to reduce, and they really need a breast lift instead. Insurance won't pay for a breast lift, so if this is true for you, be aware that you'll have to pay for the lift surgery yourself. Even if your breasts are sagging, hanging, and feeling heavy, you might not have enough breast tissue for reduction surgery.

Insurance companies generally won't cover the procedure as medically necessary unless the patient has a minimum number of grams of tissue per breast to be removed. Even if there's enough breast tissue to perform the surgery, there might not be enough removed for the insurance company to pay for it as a medical necessity—in other words, the insurance company might determine that breast surgery is cosmetic. Usually, prior authorization is required before proceeding with surgery unless patients are paying for the procedures themselves. After performing reduction surgery for years and interacting with insurance companies, I have a sense for what they'll cover and what they'll likely deny. When examining a potential reduction patient, if I don't think a reduction is medically necessary based on my experience, I'll give the patient a cosmetic-procedure quote. Again, you need to be prepared to pay for the surgery if your insurance company denies coverage because it decides the surgery isn't medically necessary. Not all surgeons accept insurance for this procedure and, therefore, are self-pay only. So, ask your insurance company for a list of plastic surgeons who accept your insurance.

Furthermore, some insurance companies might deny a reduction if you don't provide evidence of medical necessity. This means you might have to prove that you tried—and exhausted—nonsurgical options such as physical therapy or chiropractor visits related to heavy breasts.

Surgery: The surgery typically takes one and a half to three hours, and most surgeries are either outpatient or inpatient procedures with the patient under general anesthesia. The degree of breast droopiness determines the type of incisions your surgeon will make. Depending on the degree of laxity of your skin, you will require a short vertical-scar reduction or a full anchor-incision-pattern reduction. Your surgeon will try to ensure that scars are as inconspicuous as possible.

After breast-reduction surgery: Swelling and bruising occur after any surgery to varying degrees. As with other breast surgeries, the swelling tends to peak at about forty-eight hours, then rapidly decreases. About 50 percent of swelling is gone by the end of the first few weeks, but during this early period, your breasts will appear larger than their final size because of the swelling. Most swelling is gone by six to eight weeks and is barely perceptible by six months.

BEFORE   **AFTER**

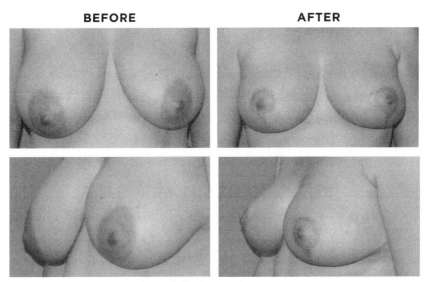

Before and after breast reduction surgery.

NOT JUST FOR WOMEN

Men with gynecomastia (enlarged breasts in men) are often seeking breast reduction. Whether they are embarrassed to go to the beach and taking off their shirt, or they are younger and are bullied, I can reduce the breast tissue from gynecomastia and help patients gain their confidence back. This is done in an outpatient setting and usually requires a combination of liposuction and direct removal of tissue. Sometimes no tissue is removed and liposuction alone is enough. If an incision is required, it is usually placed along the border of the areola where it can be hidden after healing. In some cases, surgical drains will be left for one week. You can expect to wear a compression garment for six weeks.

BEFORE **AFTER**

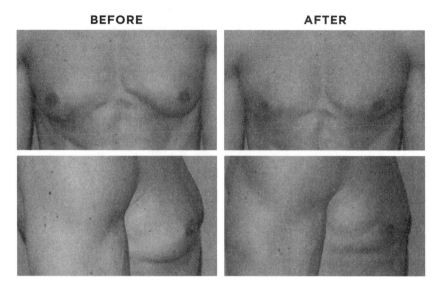

Before and after breast reduction for a patient with gynecomastia.

NIPPLE/AREOLA SURGERY

The nipple and areola make up one of the most cosmetic aspects of the breast, and patients who have excessively large areolas, inverted nipples, or nipples that look puffy can be embarrassed and unhappy with their appearance. A surgeon can easily correct these nipple or areola problems in a relatively minor surgery, often done in the office under local or twilight anesthesia, or as part of any breast procedure (augmentation, reduction, or lift). The next short sections discuss the three nipple conditions that surgery can correct.

INVERTED NIPPLES

Inward-pointing nipples (or inverted) are common, and about 2 percent of women have this problem on one or both breasts. Inverted nipples can result from a narrow nipple base, excessively short milk ducts, or from scarring of the milk ducts (after a milk-duct infection, for example). In mild cases, the nipples tend to invert when stimulated by cold or touch, but they're usually in the normal position. In most cases surgical correction is required. The milk ducts beneath the nipple are severed to release the nipple, and dissolvable sutures are placed to hold the nipple out. Breastfeeding function is completely lost, while sensation is preserved.

ELONGATED NIPPLES

Many patients suffer from long nipples and simply want them to be shortened. This can be embarrassing for patients who wear bathing suits or are braless beneath a t-shirt. There is a very simple procedure that can be done in the office under local anesthesia or during another breast procedure in the operating room. It requires removing some of the nipple tissue from the tip of the nipple and closing it with sutures. It will heal and the resulting appearance will be a shorter nipple that does not project as much as it once did.

AREOLA REDUCTION

Areolas come in all shapes and sizes, but some women are concerned if their areolas are too large, possibly associated with large breasts. Areola-reduction surgery reduces the amount of darker pigmented skin. Besides reducing the areola size, this procedure can slightly tighten the breast and lift the nipple higher. An areola reduction alone can be performed under local anesthesia in the surgeon's office in some cases. Most are performed along with other breast procedures, such as reduction or lift (performed in the operating room under general anesthesia).

Another condition can occur when one nipple/areola complex is lower or higher than the other. This can be corrected by raising the lower nipple/areola complex to match the other breast's nipple/areola position.

Some patients have very large nipples that may be reduced under local anesthesia alone or done in the operating room while asleep for another procedure. Part of the excess tissue is removed, the wound sutured closed, and the resulting nipple is much smaller.

PUFFY AREOLAS

Puffy areolas occur when the skin of the areola isn't as thick as the surrounding skin, and the underlying breast tissue pushes through, causing fullness under the areola. Puffy areolas are often seen in women with tuberous breast deformity (cone shaped). Procedures to flatten out the puffiness reduce both the underlying breast tissue and the size of the areola. The surgery shouldn't affect breastfeeding, because the milk ducts are still intact, and milk flow is uninterrupted, assuming there were no problems before surgery.

Initial consultation: The surgeon will discuss your situation, describe the procedure to correct it, and discuss scarring. For inverted nipples, the procedure severs the milk ducts, causing permanent loss of the ability to breastfeed. You should talk about this in your consultation, and consider whether you can live with that result. The surgeon should also tell you that even a good procedure might not correct inverted nipples completely, and that they can recur, albeit rarely. For areola surgery, it depends on whether the areola is being reduced in size or if the areola tissue beneath is being removed. Both require an incision around the areola to complete and when removing tissue for puffy areolas, milk ducts can be injured permanently as well.

Surgery: Nipple and areola surgery can be performed together or separate. The surgery takes about an hour and typically may require local anesthesia or general anesthesia depending on what is being done. For nipple surgery, the area is anesthetized and a small portion of tissue is removed and sutured closed. For areola surgery, the surgeon will remove some of the darker skin on the outer edge of the areola and then draw in the normal skin to surround the new edge. Permanent stitching, placed deep in the tissue, if used, will keep the areola from widening during recovery. Dissolving stitches retain the smaller areola diameter as the skin heals.

After nipple/areola surgery: Nipple or areola procedures result in little downtime if done alone, because they're not as invasive as other, more complex breast procedures. You'll feel some discomfort and have some swelling and bruising for a few days. The same lifting restrictions are in place with any scar such as no lifting of more than twenty pounds for six weeks. Cardiac-type exercise is generally re-introduced after one month.

BREAST RECONSTRUCTION

Women who have breast cancer can undergo tumor removal (resection by lumpectomy) or have one or both breasts removed (mastectomy), and they have several breast-reconstruction options. Reconstruction typically restores a sense of wholeness and helps patients continue with their lives. If you are having a lumpectomy and are large breasted, you may simply have a breast reduction as your reconstructive procedure. Once the lump is removed, the plastic surgeon will finish by reducing that breast as they normally would do in any breast reduction. Both breasts would be addressed at the same time. I perform this operation on a regular basis. The surgeon can often perform the first stage of reconstruction at the same time as the mastectomy procedure, but might need to change the plan depending on whether the patient needs radiation treatment right away. Plastic surgeons work closely with the team of doctors (surgical oncologist, medical oncologist, and radiation oncologist) to plan the type of reconstruction that's best. Breast reconstruction isn't for everyone, though. It might take more than one operation and could take up to a year to complete. Some women decide not to have reconstruction and are very comfortable with their decision.

Initial consultation: You'll discuss the variety of reconstructive operations that fall into two main categories: procedures that borrow your own tissue from one part of the body, or strictly implant-based reconstruction with saline or silicone implants. You should leave your breast-reconstruction consultation with no doubts or unanswered questions. Your desires and goals, lifestyle, overall health, body type, and what the oncologic team determines is your safest course of action will all determine the best procedures for you.

Expectations are another important part of the discussion. It's crucial to have realistic expectations about restoration surgery, because it won't restore the breasts to their original look or feel. They might look better—even great—but they won't feel the same. They'll look awesome in clothing, and you'll look normal. But when you take your shirt off, they won't resemble the breasts you had before the mastectomy, because they're made from muscle, skin, and implants only. This is an incredibly hard discussion to have with my mastectomy patients. I try to make them feel comfortable with the idea that the reconstruction can restore their femininity when they're clothed and going about their daily lives. But sometimes, the nipple and areola are gone because of the cancer. Certain patients will have nipple-sparing mastectomies, depending on the cancer location. Other solutions are to build a nipple followed by areolar tattoo, or to simply tattoo nipples and areolas on the reconstructed breasts, and they'll look fantastic. I try to prepare these patients as best I can for that result, and managing their expectations is probably the hardest part of the whole breast-reconstruction experience.

Surgery: The length of surgery varies greatly and can often take one to three hours for something like an implant/expander reconstruction or up to six hours for a more complicated reconstruction.

- Implant-based reconstruction: Your surgeon will generally use the same mastectomy incisions that your surgical oncologist made to remove the breast—whether performing the reconstruction at the same time as the mastectomy (immediate reconstruction) or weeks, months, or years later (delayed reconstruction). You'll have additional scars if using your own tissues for reconstruction, and your surgeon will discuss this with you at your consultation. After reconstruction is complete with implants, there may be the need for additional soft-tissue coverage to even out both sides. I use fat transfer, using the body's own fat like a filler. I liposuction it from one part of the body and then re-inject it into the skin envelope of the breast to fill areas that need contouring.

- Implant/expander reconstruction: If the patient is a candidate, the surgeon can go directly to placing the final implants at the time of mastectomy. If for some reason that is not possible, a two-step process may be utilized. In the first stage, your surgeon places a tissue expander underneath the chest muscle (pectoralis). The implant is filled with saline to inflate it gradually over several weeks, usually eight to twelve weeks in weekly appointments in the office after all incisions have healed. A second surgery, scheduled after the skin has expanded adequately, involves removing the expander and replacing it with a permanent implant (saline or silicone). Patients having radiation won't undergo this second stage for at least six months after completing radiation treatment, because the skin's blood supply and elasticity need time to recover from radiation damage. Your surgeon will discuss the many variations of this process with you at your consultation.

BEFORE   **AFTER**

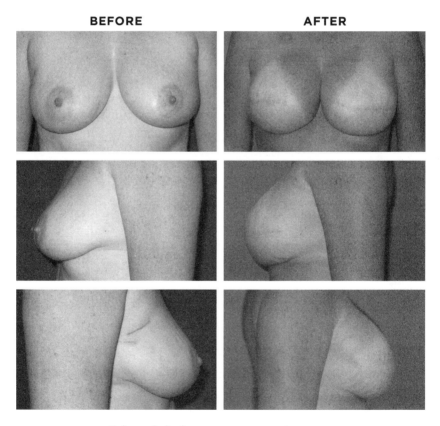

Before and after breast cancer reconstruction surgery.

CHAPTER 7

Body Procedures

At some point in your life—whether from having kids or simply from aging—you might find that your flat tummy and curvy, contoured thighs just aren't what they used to be. You might even have extra skin and fatty tissue on your upper arms. So, you exercise and follow strict meal plans, and you exercise and diet and exercise some more, but the fat just won't budge. It seems that no matter what you do, the tummy bulge, jiggly thighs, and flabby arms stubbornly resist exercise and meal planning. Body procedures such as liposuction, lifts, or a combination of both (also called body contouring) can help get rid of skin and fat.

LIPOSUCTION

Patients want liposuction most often for the tummy, outer and inner thighs, flanks and bra line. Liposuction surgery can help you achieve a sleeker, more toned look by removing modest amounts of fat in targeted areas, leaving you with natural curves that complement your frame. It's not a weight-loss solution, though—it's a body-sculpting procedure that can eliminate stubborn areas of fat that haven't responded well to diet and exercise, and any significant weight fluctuations after your surgery can reverse some of the procedure's benefits. For some patients, liposuction is a debulking procedure to make clothing fit more comfortably.

Initial consultation: You and your surgeon will discuss the areas you'd like to treat, your options, the likely outcomes, and the risks and any potential complications, along with details of how to prepare for surgery and what to expect as you heal. You'll probably look at liposuction before-and-after photos to help you develop realistic expectations for the results. If you still need to lose weight, your surgeon might advise you to do so before liposuction to better define your trouble areas and improve your overall results. You might also discuss using traditional or ultrasonic liposuction, depending on which options your surgeon offers. Both options use a small tube (cannula) to suction out your stubborn fat deposits. Your surgeon will also discuss whether you could have residual loose skin after the procedure.

Surgery: The liposuction procedure takes about one to two hours, depending on how many areas you want treated. The procedure can be outpatient or inpatient under twilight or general anesthesia. The morning of surgery, your physician will mark the liposuction sites and answer any last-minute questions you might have. The surgeon will make one or two incisions per treatment area (only a few millimeters long), hidden as inconspicuously as possible in the natural folds of your skin.

After liposuction surgery: Most patients can go home the day of surgery. You can expect the greatest amount of swelling in two to four days after surgery. This is normal during healing, and the swelling and bruising will begin to decrease quickly so that at two weeks, most bruising will be gone, and at six to eight weeks, almost all swelling will be gone. Most patients feel well enough to return to normal activities after a few days, but you should avoid strenuous activity until your physician clears you to do so.

TUMMY TUCK

A tummy tuck (abdominoplasty) is a surgical procedure for removing extra skin and fat in the abdomen. A tummy tuck also involves tightening the six-pack muscles that often stretch out and bulge in women who've had children, or in overweight patients who have lost a lot of weight, resulting in a flatter, tighter tummy. The procedure can include liposuction to blend the surrounding areas. You might be a good candidate for a tummy tuck if you're healthy and your weight is stable, but you have excess loose skin and fat around the abdomen. If you have stretch marks, a tummy tuck can remove most of them along with the extra skin.

Initial consultation: Your first discussion in your consultation should be about where you are in your weight-loss journey. If you're within five to ten pounds of your ideal weight, you're probably a good candidate for surgery. But if you're outside those parameters, you might need to delay the procedure until you meet your weight goal. This is particularly true for people who carry visceral fat (the fat surrounding your organs) that might contribute to abdominal bulge, even after muscle repair. Pregnancy is another consideration, and patients who want more kids should postpone tummy-tuck surgery until after the last pregnancy. The surgeon will discuss expectations, because some patients have an unrealistic picture of how flat the surgery can make the tummy. Other topics for the consultation are incisions and scars, and the possibility that the procedure might not remove all stretch marks.

Surgery: The operation takes two to three hours, depending on whether you're also having liposuction with the procedure. Most surgeries are performed either outpatient or inpatient, under general anesthesia. The surgeon can hide the incision in the panty line in most cases. The length of the incision depends on how much extra skin you have, but it usually runs from one hip bone to the other. You'll also have an incision around your navel, but this incision is usually imperceptible once it heals. There is also a "mini" tummy tuck, which does not require an incision around the naval and is for women who just need skin below the belly button removed.

After tummy-tuck surgery: Your surgeon will place one or two drains underneath the abdominal tissue that had to be elevated from the underlying muscles. These drains help prevent fluid collection that can hinder the healing process, and they're typically removed from one to two weeks after surgery. Swelling and bruising can occur to varying degrees, peaking at about forty-eight hours and then rapidly decreasing. By the end of the first few weeks, 50 percent of the swelling will be gone, and most swelling will diminish by six to eight weeks. Almost all the swelling will be gone by six months. Any remaining swelling is almost imperceptible.

THIGH LIFT

A thigh lift could be a good procedure for you if you're dissatisfied with the shape of your thighs, especially after a dramatic weight loss. Patients who've had massive weight loss from diet and exercise or bariatric weight-loss surgery commonly have excess skin. The procedure, usually performed after massive weight loss, removes excess, sagging skin of the inner thighs to alter the shape of the thigh and create a more desirable contour. It can also fix naturally sagging thigh tissue. Liposuction can treat fat by itself, without excess skin. Combining liposuction with body-lift procedures can treat the outer thighs.

Initial consultation: The surgeon will ask you about your goals and discuss which parts of your thigh bother you, such as the area from the hip to the knees or in the groin area. The biggest areas of discussion will be about the procedure, the type of incisions needed, and the resulting scars. To tighten and lift the thigh, the incision in the groin area sometimes extends down the inside of the thigh, resulting in long scars that look like hockey sticks. If you can't live with such scars, you shouldn't have the procedure. Expectations, again, are important to discuss because thigh lifts won't last forever. Unfortunately, when you stand upright, gravity wins, and minor sagginess recurs with time.

Surgery: The procedure takes about two hours. Your surgeon can combine it with other procedures, which would take longer. Most surgeries are in an outpatient setting or inpatient in an operating suite with the patient under general anesthesia. Incisions can extend all the way down to your inner-knee region, depending on how much skin the surgeon plans to remove. The incisions can be entirely in the groin crease in some cases. Thigh lifts are safe as an outpatient procedure, and most patients can go home the same day.

After thigh-lift surgery: Sometimes your surgeon will place drains under the skin in each leg and remove them one to two weeks after surgery. Wraps placed around each leg from the toes to the thigh region will help control postoperative swelling, which peaks at about forty-eight hours, and then rapidly decreases to 50 percent by the end of the first few weeks, is mostly gone by six to eight weeks, and is almost completely gone by six months. Sutures are typically dissolvable, and the surgeon will usually remove drains in seven to ten days after surgery, but they could be left in place for longer than ten days if they're putting out too much fluid. This is rare, though.

ARM LIFT

You might be an ideal candidate for an arm lift if you have excess skin and fat on your upper arms. The procedure, often performed after massive weight loss, removes excess sagging skin and fat from the arms. Most patients need a combination of liposuction and skin removal.

Initial consultation: Your surgeon will determine what you like and don't like about your arms, usually extra skin or bulkiness, and not just on the backs of the arms, but sometimes extending into the armpit area beside the breast. The possibility of needing a two-stage procedure is another topic for patients who have excessively large arms. The surgeon will also discuss the need for drains, though in my practice, I do a drainless procedure, so patients don't have to deal with them.

Scarring is the most important topic in the consultation. Scars can be inside the arm or sometimes directly down the backside of the arm, and your surgeon should discuss the pros and cons of each. Most patients end up with well-healed scars. Extremities potentially have the least-favorable scarring outcomes of anywhere on the body, because they're the highest area of tension. That said, I make sure I do not over resect tissue in an effort to create the least amount of tension possible, resulting in flat, thin and pretty scars. You may start using silicone-based treatments several weeks after surgery once the incisions are completely closed. Lasers and scar injections are also an option for treating scars that become too thick.

Surgery: The operation takes about two hours, but it can take longer if combined with other procedures. Most surgeries are in an outpatient setting or inpatient with the patient under general anesthesia. Incisions are usually on the inner portion of the arm and can extend from the elbow into the armpit, depending on how much skin the surgeon has to remove. Arm lifts are safe as an outpatient procedure, and most patients can go home the same day.

After arm-lift surgery: You'll have bandages from the wrists all the way to the top of your arms to help decrease swelling. Compression will be required for six weeks for best results. You can remove these wraps when you take a shower, but will need to put them back on after. Compression sleeves will give you the best result because it helps to contour the arms. The surgeon will remove any surgical drains if used in seven to ten days after surgery and can do it in the office.

BEFORE   **AFTER**

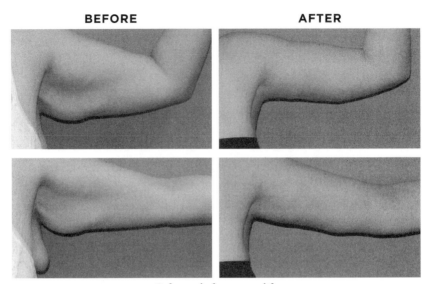

Before and after an arm lift.

CHAPTER 8

Gluteal Procedures

Some women have a shapely butt, and some don't. Some have a butt and want a fuller one. Others have laxity from aging, weight loss, or gravity that they'd like to tighten up in ways that working out won't accomplish. Gluteal procedures can fix these problems and create butts that are fuller, more curvy, and more perky.

GLUTEAL AUGMENTATION (BUTT LIFT)

Women who had several children might be interested in restoring their butts to how they looked before having children. Butt lift surgery lifts and tightens loose, hanging skin on the buttocks and upper outer thighs by removing the excess skin from the lower-back area that has stretched. The goal of this surgery is to return the body to a more normal appearance after a loss of skin elasticity caused by aging, pregnancy, or extreme weight loss. This procedure is different from a Brazilian butt lift, which uses injections of the patient's own fat to increase projection and create a lifting effect, and to contour for a more aesthetic appearance. Surgeons can combine a butt lift with fat injections or use the patient's own skin folded inward to augment for a full, round shape. A butt lift's purpose isn't to remove significant fat deposits, but it can remove small amounts of fat along with excess skin.

Many people ask if a butt lift will eliminate cellulite or stretch marks. It won't get rid of cellulite, but it will tighten the area and contour it for a more youthful shape. The lift can remove stretch marks only where skin is removed. The outcome will be different for each patient, but generally, stretch marks and cellulite tend to improve greatly after surgery.

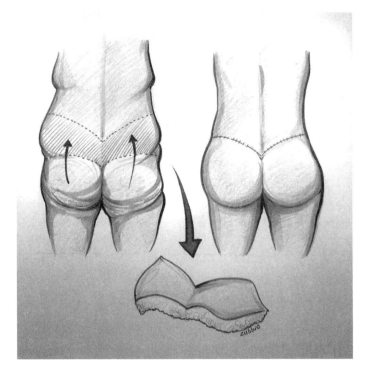

Credit: Christian Subbio, MD, board certified plastic surgeon

Initial consultation: Your surgeon will discuss whether you're a good candidate for a butt lift based on your weight, which should be stable or nearly ideal before even considering this procedure. You'll discuss expectations for the results regarding any stretch marks or cellulite you might have.

Surgery: In this procedure, your surgeon removes excess skin and repositions the surrounding tissue to create a more youthful and pleasing body contour. Incisions to remove excess skin and pull the remaining skin tighter can be in several places, depending on your needs: at the top of the buttocks extending around to the outer hips or, in rare cases, under the butt cheeks in the gluteal crease. The procedure requires drains and a compression garment to reduce swelling and tighten the skin. Liposuction can further contour the buttock area or thighs if needed.

After butt lift surgery: The buttocks will feel very tight for several days after surgery. In the first few days, you'll feel most comfortable lying flat, but will be able to sit upright during the next several days. You might feel occasional twinges of discomfort at first, and it will take several months for the butt to feel normal again. Temporary numbness is common, especially just below the incision. The scar often becomes redder a few weeks after surgery but begins to fade over the course of a year. The scar will never disappear completely, but its appearance is usually very satisfactory. It could take the scar as long as twelve months to reach its final appearance, and it might require laser treatments to improve appearance and quality.

BRAZILIAN BUTT LIFT

The Brazilian Butt Lift procedure transfers fat to the butt that's lipo-suctioned from other parts of the body to create a fuller and lifting effect. Many women love the Brazilian Butt Lift's round, projecting buttocks and more contoured, lifted appearance. Surgeons liposuc-tion fat for transfer from the so-called love handles, the abdomen, the back, or other areas if needed. A beautiful result can be obtained in one surgery, but sometimes touch-up procedures are required. Gluteal implants can be used, but often more surgeries are required to fix drastic problems that can occur, and this is why I prefer the fat-transfer procedure to implants. However, implants or Sculptra injec-tions might be the only option for women who don't have enough fat for transfer.

Initial consultation: Your surgeon will discuss possible areas from which to liposuction fat for transfer. An important issue to discuss is the possibility of needing skin resection at the same time of fat transfer, because fat alone may not lift the butt completely. Also, about 60 percent of transferred fat cells will live and about 40 percent will die, so you might need touch-up procedures later, however a vast majority of patients only require one procedure. Postoperative care is a big topic in the discussion, because patients can't sit normally for about six weeks and will have to sleep on their tummies.

Surgery: Your surgeon will perform liposuction first to harvest the fat needed to transfer to the butt. In the transfer procedure, the surgeon injects fat into the buttocks through several small incisions. Typically, the surgeon will overfill the area because of normal expected loss within the first six weeks. The limit to how much can be placed is relative to the laxity of the skin.

After fat transfer surgery: After surgery, the patient wears a compression garment, which helps hold the shape. Most of the fat that's going to die will do so in the first six weeks, and the fat that remains alive after about six weeks should be permanent. Discomfort from this surgery usually subsides quickly after seven to ten days. The patient has to sleep on the stomach for six weeks after surgery and avoid sitting as much as possible for the first couple of weeks. You will purchase a special pillow to help keep pressure off of the buttocks for the first six weeks.

ABOUT GLUTEAL IMPLANTS

Gluteal implants aren't my favorite way to achieve gluteal enhancement, so I don't do them. Either the Brazilian Butt Lift or a gluteal lift is a better way to produce lasting results with less chance of complications. There are just too many disaster stories about infected gluteal implants, and they can rotate out of position because people sit on them. They can even extrude, meaning the implant pushes through the skin over time and becomes exposed, thus requiring immediate removal.

CHAPTER 9

The Mommy Makeover

When you give birth, it wreaks havoc on your body—no two ways about it. Pregnancy can dramatically change the quality of your skin and muscle tone. Women come into my office all the time and tell me things like, "Okay, I've had my last kid, and now I hate my tummy; I have a bunch of extra skin, I have stretch marks, and my breasts are saggy and deflated." These women don't feel good in a swimming suit—they panic at the thought of putting one on, because their bodies just don't look the same anymore; they don't feel like themselves. They come in to talk about what plastic surgery can do to help them get back the bodies they had before having children, and we have just the thing: the Mommy Makeover. It's a group of procedures—breast surgeries, liposuction, arm and tummy tucks, gluteal augmentation, and even vaginal rejuvenation—that can repair a lot of the damage that pregnancy causes to the body.

A Mommy Makeover is something you can do for yourself that really has positive effects—huge effects, in fact, in ways you can't imagine. I've had patients come back to me crying because they're so happy and never felt so alive, and they look amazing in clothes they never thought they could wear again. Their breasts now have the shape they want, they fit into their favorite dresses again, they have cleavage again, their tummies are flat again, and all the extra skin and most of their stretch marks are gone. They're wearing bikinis, shorts, and short-sleeved shirts again. Mommy Makeover procedures are life changing for these patients.

You can have most of the Mommy Makeover procedures done at the same time, if you're healthy and your surgeon decides that it's safe. You get your results all at once, go through recovery from all of the procedures just once, and get your rejuvenated body in one shot. It's no wonder so many women are in tears for good reasons after having these procedures.

MOMMY MAKEOVER EXPECTATIONS

A Mommy Makeover can do many things for you, including:

- making you feel better about yourself and your body again

- making your clothes fit better again

- tightening your abdominal muscles and removes excess skin and soft tissue to help restore your prepregnancy figure

- reshaping and contouring your body by removing fat deposits that diet and exercise just can't seem to conquer

- lifting your breasts and adding volume back to restore them to their youthful, prepregnancy look

- slimming, tightening, and shaping your arms so you no longer have excess skin

- slimming and contouring your thighs so you can wear short skirts and shorts again

- repairing vaginal damage so you can enjoy sex the way you did before you had kids, and

- restoring confidence during intimate times.

A Mommy Makeover can do only so much, though. As life changing as a Mommy Makeover can be, you need to have realistic expectations for these procedures, just like any other plastic-surgery procedure. Here are some things a Mommy Makeover won't do:

- Return you to the *exact* body you had before pregnancy.

- Get rid of all your stretch marks.

- Make you lose weight.

- Get you a partner if you're single or save a failing marriage.

- Solve your home problems.

And on a slightly different note, there's one more very important thing that the Mommy Makeover won't do: it won't keep you from continuing a healthy lifestyle with good eating habits and exercise.

However, even though this makeover won't return your body to exactly how it was before pregnancy, nor suddenly turn you into a fashion model, it will definitely fix many of the changes resulting from pregnancy and give you renewed confidence in your body. The important thing is to have realistic expectations about what is possible for you. If you can do that, you'll be very happy with your makeover results.

IS THE TIME RIGHT?

After reading about what the Mommy Makeover can do and has done for many women, you might look in the mirror and decide that you want to have the procedures right now—like tomorrow, or this afternoon. But you need to consider the following three things before getting really serious about this surgery:

1. Are you going to have more kids?

2. Are you still breastfeeding?

3. Are you at an ideal body weight?

If you want to have more kids, you should wait to have the surgery until you're sure you're done having children. Another pregnancy would restretch the muscles that a tummy tuck tightens, and you'd be right back to where you were before. Similarly, if you're still breastfeeding, breast surgery has to wait three to six months after you're finished nursing to allow the tissue to return to its more native state so your surgeon can perform an accurate assessment to determine the right procedure and size for you.

VAGINAL REJUVENATION

You've already read about all of the procedures that typically make up the Mommy Makeover except for one: vaginal rejuvenation. Procedures for vaginal rejuvenation are becoming more popular, usually as part of a Mommy Makeover. Giving birth can stretch out the vagina and weaken the muscles, and it just doesn't feel like it used to feel—most women say that it doesn't feel as tight as it was. Several things result from this, not the least of which is that sex isn't as enjoyable as it used to be. Often, there is excess labial tissue that needs to be removed. The internal tightness that many women lose makes having sex less enjoyable, and for those cases, tightening procedures using a laser or surgery can help. Childbirth can also result in urological issues, but you should see a urogynecologist to address these issues. A urogynecologist is a physician with special training in urology, gynecology, and obstetrics who evaluates and treats non-cancerous conditions of the female pelvic organs and their supporting muscles and tissues.

As with all of the Mommy-Makeover procedures, you should wait until you're finished having children before having any vaginal-rejuvenation surgery.

There are two main procedures involved in vaginal rejuvenation.

TIGHTENING PROCEDURES

These procedures tighten the inner and outer muscles and structures of the vagina to enhance vaginal muscle tone, strength, and control. Most commonly, laser or radiofrequency waves apply a small amount of heat to the internal lining of the vagina, causing that area to tighten by contracting the collagen and elastin in the tissue. It's a simple, straightforward, minimally invasive procedure; and it's relatively painless, takes less than a half hour to perform, and leads to no downtime. Most patients typically need more than one treatment. However, these treatments can be ineffective for patients whose vaginal muscles are extremely lax, and a surgical option is required for them. The surgery removes extra skin from the backside of the vagina and brings separated muscles together.

LABIAL REDUCTION

Some women are born with too much tissue on the labia—either the small, inner lips (minor labia) or the larger, outer lips (the major labia)—and some have it because of childbirth. They don't like how it looks in a bathing suit, or they're embarrassed with how it looks when they're intimate with their partner. Some women have a lot of extra skin on only one side, which doesn't usually cause any physical problems, but it just doesn't look right to them, and they want both sides to match. Labial-reduction surgery reduces the volume of labial tissue to correct these problems. Sometimes the major labia lack volume and, in those cases, fat transfer can be performed to restore balance to this area.

PREPARING FOR A MOMMY MAKEOVER

You'll get the best results from a Mommy Makeover if you're within ten pounds of your ideal body weight when you have the procedures. This is really important. I have turned a patient away for surgery because she was still overweight. She had already lost a lot of weight and wanted her arms and tummy fixed. I was excited for her for successfully losing fifty pounds (I mean, that's amazing), but she wasn't there yet. She needed to lose a lot more weight before she'd be ready for the procedure for lots of reasons. Above all, it isn't safe to put someone with a high body mass index under anesthesia. But related to the makeover, she just wasn't going to get a good result until she lost the weight—because if I took out her extra skin and she lost even more weight, she would just have more extra skin again.

Making sure that you're near your ideal weight is just one of the things you'll need to do to prepare for a Mommy Makeover. Here's the list:

- Get your diet and lifestyle in order so you can lose enough weight to have a great result. If you still need to lose more weight, do it before the surgery.

- Talk with your family and friends about the surgery, why you want to have it, and what you expect from it (see chapter 3).

- Be sure you have someone to help you with the kids after surgery. You'll be limited on how much weight you can lift for about six weeks (no more than twenty pounds), so you'll need help. Planning for this ahead of time makes recovery better, because you won't stress out so much about not being able to take care of your kids.

- Prepare for your consultation by being ready to set priorities if you can't afford all the procedures you want. Decide which things are the most important to you.

Plastic surgery can't replace good, healthy habits like an exercise routine and a healthy meal plan. A Mommy Makeover will take care of the physical problems that healthy eating and exercise alone can't fix—it can tighten or remove loose skin, rejuvenate deflated breasts, and tighten the abdominal wall muscles. But it's up to you to do what you can first to achieve the best results, before having any Mommy Makeover procedures, and these habits will also help you maintain results after surgery.

CHAPTER 10

Procedures after Bariatric Weight-Loss Surgery

Bariatric weight-loss surgery uses several techniques to reduce the size of the stomach to prevent patients from eating as much as they used to eat. Obese patients who undergo bariatric surgery to lose weight can have remarkable results, losing from 100 to 175 pounds or more. Try to imagine the volume of fat that weighs between 100 and 175 pounds. That much volume really stretches out the skin in time, so people who lose that much fat have incredibly stretched-out, saggy skin on the face, neck, breasts (both men and women), arms, the backs of the arms, the armpit area, the abdomen, hips, thighs, and the butt. Literally, losing that much weight makes everything sag and deflate. In many cases, such a massive weight loss destroys the quality of collagen and elastic fibers in the skin. Those patients usually want skin-reducing procedures such as the following:

- **Arm lift:** The surgery removes all the extra skin.

- **Thigh lift:** The surgeon removes extra skin and lifts the thigh to support and tighten it for a better appearance.

- **Tummy tuck:** The standard or fleur-de-lis tummy-tuck procedure addresses the loose, stretched-out muscles from being overweight, along with removing excess skin.

- **Circumferential body lift (or simply body lift):** This is a major procedure for abdominal weight-loss patients. The incision starts in the front at the pubic bone for a tummy tuck, and then continues all the way around to the back above the butt. On the front side, the surgeon performs the traditional tummy-tuck tightening procedure, then flips the patient over onto his or her tummy, removes all the extra skin from the lower back area, and lifts the thighs and the butt.

- **Bra line lift:** This is for patients who have a massive amount of extra skin in the bra strap area on the upper back. Patients who want this don't care about a scar on the back—they just want the surgeon to cut out all of that tissue on their upper back. Sometimes, this lift simply removes whatever loose skin is in the back area.

Patients who want multiple procedures should be ready to have more than one surgery, because it's not safe to do too many procedures at the same time. I often stage these procedures over several months. I might do the breast and arms in one surgery, then let the patient recover for a month or two. After that recovery period, I do the tummy and thighs. For the circumferential body lift, I prefer doing it in stages because of safety issues and the risks of poor scarring. When patients undergo the tummy-tuck part of the procedure, I want them to hunch forward a little bit during recovery to keep pressure off that incision, because tension is one of the factors that causes poor scarring. If I do the back part of the body lift at the same time, then the patients would be putting more tension on the back scar while trying to take it off the front scar—they can't win either way. So I might do the front tummy part in one surgery and the back part in another. But the front and back *can* be done together if needed.

READY FOR SURGERY?

Now that you've learned about the various plastic-surgery body procedures, I'll tell you what to expect from surgery before, during, and after the procedure, with a particular focus on self-care after the procedure to ensure lasting results.

Everything You Need to Know About Surgery — Before, During, and After

Some of my patients have been lucky: They managed to go through their entire lives without needing any kind of surgery or hospitalization. So, when they're facing their elective plastic-surgery procedures, they have no idea what to expect and don't know anything about what a patient experiences before, during, and after surgery. A big part of my job is to make sure that patients have plenty of information, guidance, and instructions about surgery and what they need to do, as well as what they're going to experience from start to finish. Part 3 covers the typical information I give to my patients so that they're fully prepared for their surgery and recovery.

Never, *ever* stop medications until instructed to do so by the medical professional looking after you.

Never, *ever* stop medications until instructed to do so by the medical professional looking after you.

I like to prepare my patients for surgery as soon as they've decided to have it. The following are important steps that I want my patients to take right away to help ensure a smooth, successful surgery and recovery:

- **Stop smoking or using any nicotine products.** Nicotine reduces circulation to the skin and delays healing by restricting small blood vessels, whether you smoke cigarettes, chew nicotine gum, suck on nicotine lozenges, or allow nicotine to enter your body in any other way. You must stop for a minimum of four weeks before surgery and stay away from nicotine for a minimum of four weeks after surgery. (Tip of the day: This would be a great time to quit if you're going to be off the stuff for two months anyway. Think about it in the context of a completely new you.)

- **Stop taking aspirin.** If you take aspirin, you should stop taking it one week before surgery, but only with the approval of your medical professionals. Use medications containing acetaminophen instead, such as Tylenol.

- **Stop taking herbal supplements and blood thinners.** For the same reason, you don't want to take anything that will make it harder for your blood to coagulate. Many herbal supplements thin the blood, so you should check with your medical professional before stopping any medications.

- **Limit vitamin E.** Higher doses of vitamin E can increase the risk of bleeding, because it can counteract the coagulation properties of other substances, such as vitamin K.

- **Fill prescriptions before the day of surgery.** Your surgeon might give you prescriptions before your surgery day. It's a good idea to fill them as soon as you get them so you don't forget, and you'll have them as needed when you get home after surgery. Even more important, you won't have to stop on the way home after surgery. You'll want to just get home and start your recovery at that point.

• **Tell your doctor if you have any sign of a cold or other infection a week before surgery.** Your surgeon might want to postpone your procedure if you show any signs of a cold, flu, or especially an upper respiratory infection because such illnesses could increase the likelihood of experiencing breathing problems under anesthesia. Likewise, having any active infection when you're facing implant surgery increases your risks for an implant infection. Postponing your surgery would surely be disappointing, but your safety is your surgeon's number-one concern.

• **Again, never stop taking medications from your medical professional unless instructed otherwise.** For instance, if your medical provider has you taking necessary blood thinners that are essential to your health, let your surgeon know, and continue taking them normally.

INPATIENT OR OUTPATIENT PROCEDURE?

Your surgeon can perform some procedures on an outpatient basis, but others require you to spend at least one night in a surgical facility where staff can monitor you. The type of procedure isn't necessarily the deciding factor. It depends on the particular patient, because all patients are different and have different medical histories and backgrounds. Your surgeon will decide whether an inpatient or outpatient procedure is right for you based on clinical judgment. Some patients just need overnight monitoring after having an anesthetic for four, six, or eight hours. Others who have a medical condition, like a history of seizures or minor cardiac history, would likely have an inpatient procedure so staff can monitor them to make sure the condition doesn't cause problems after surgery. Surgeons follow some clear guidelines for identifying and predicting which patients are, or are likely to be, at high risk for non-cardiac surgery.

I require some patients to stay overnight, because they're having so many procedures at one time that it's just not safe for them to be home alone the first night. We usually discuss this at their consultation. An example of a patient I'd require to stay overnight would be someone having a breast augmentation and lift, a tummy tuck, and some liposuction. That can be over six hours of surgery, and in my opinion, the patient would be too uncomfortable to go home, and it could be unsafe. Your spouse, partner, or any other support person probably wouldn't be able to provide you with the competent, professional care that a recovery center's nursing staff can. However, many surgeons would allow you to go home after these procedures if they feel comfortable with your scenario.

If you're having a big enough procedure, you might even want an overnight stay, despite the extra cost. If you have four kids at home and their dad has to take care of them, who's going to take care of you? Frankly, you won't want the kids hanging around after the surgery, and you'll need a night of peace. Staying at an overnight care facility, even for just the first night, can give you a quiet environment so that you can rest and start your recovery. The nursing staff can give you pain and nausea medication, change your dressings, and give you ice packs for the swelling and bruising. Really, it's a bit of pampering and TLC before you go home the next day, so think about it.

If you've never had surgery—or even if you have—the next chapters explain everything you need to know about what to do before and after surgery, and what a typical surgery day is like for a plastic surgery patient.

CHAPTER 11

What to Expect Before Surgery

Your surgery day is drawing closer. This is when you, your surgeon, and the doctor's staff get busy with preparations. Whether you're having one procedure or more, you'll have some general and procedure-specific preparations to make as far out as two weeks before your surgery day. This chapter covers some of the things you can expect to happen during this time, but remember that your surgeon will give you guidance and instructions specific to you and your procedure. My own experiences with my patients are the basis for what follows.

PREOPERATIVE VISIT

Your preoperative visit is an important appointment that will start all of the activities leading up to your surgery day. You and your surgeon will finalize many details during this appointment. I usually see patients for their pre-op appointment two weeks before surgery, and I answer final questions about their specific procedure. We take preoperative photos for comparison after the procedure and for my preprocedure planning. For breast procedures, for example, I try to get the patient's vision board photos beforehand. I use the vision board (discussed in chapter 4) to guide what I'm doing in surgery, because it shows me the result the patient wants. The vision-board pictures are definitely important for me in my practice, and they've helped increase my patients' happiness and satisfaction after surgery. However, we can't use vision-board photos for other procedures, like tummy surgery and liposuction. You pretty much have what you have in those areas, and it's unrealistic to look at a photo and say, "Hey, I want my tummy to look like hers." But we do go over the expected results and make sure that everyone understands the procedure and the results clearly.

In my practice, we give patients a lot of detailed information during this appointment to help them plan ahead for their surgery and for what they'll need to do at home afterward. Some of the information is in a packet of several documents, depending on the patient's procedure. Here are some of the documents that might be in the preoperative packet—this list is just to give you an idea of the kind of information you should have before surgery:

- **Preparing for surgery document:** This document details what patients need to do in the weeks before surgery, including the day before and the day of surgery. This includes things like stopping smoking, stopping certain medications, etc.

- **Preoperative shopping list:** Patients will need a few items after surgery, some of which are specific to their procedure and others that all patients need. These common items include specific foods to eat after being under anesthesia, antibiotic ointments, gauze pads, an herbal supplement to help with bruising and swelling, and antibacterial cleanser.

- **Instructions on how to cleanse before surgery:** This document tells patients how to use surgical cleanser the day before and the day of surgery.

- **Going to the surgery center:** This document describes the operating suite, the recovery room, and the arrangements patients need to make for after their surgery.

- **As you heal:** These procedure-specific documents describe what to expect after a procedure, provide general guidelines for recovery in some cases, and answer many procedure-specific questions. We have a document for just about every procedure I perform.

I also use this time to help patients think about how they'll manage their logistics at home after the surgery and how they need to prepare their families. Some things we discuss include the following:

- **The kids:** If they have kids, who will look after them during recovery? Do they need a babysitter?

- **Where they'll recover:** Patients need to consider who's going to take care of them while they recover, particularly if they're having a major procedure.

- **Postsurgery garments:** If patients need special garments, they need to figure out where to buy them (our office is one source).

- **Postsurgery medications:** I can't stress enough how important it is to get medications before surgery, so you don't have to do it afterward.

- **Preoperative tests:** At a certain age (about age fifty), patients have to get laboratory work and an EKG before surgery, so we work together to schedule those tests. If they're younger than fifty and have medical problems that require some lab work, we schedule those tests, too. All patients should prepare for a possible delay or even cancelation of surgery if something shows up in the lab work. It's rare for that to happen, but occasionally we find a lab abnormality that we just need to address before we can safely go into surgery.

- **Finances:** Cosmetic surgery patients generally have to pay in full two weeks prior to surgery. So you'll need to make sure that your finances are in order by the time you have your preoperative appointment and be prepared to complete your payment at that time.

- **Last-minute questions and concerns:** We discuss anything you want to discuss about your procedure and recovery.

Patients spend time with my medical staff, too, discussing many presurgical details, like using the medical-grade soap to wash the night before and the morning of surgery and bringing loose, comfortable clothing with you for surgery. Any kind of breast surgery makes it hard to lift your hands over your head afterward, so breast-surgery patients need to bring button-down or zippered clothing, so they don't have to struggle to get into pullover shirts. For example, a big, comfortable flannel shirt that you can slip into and button up in the front is perfect.

We also discuss surgical drains and their care. I discuss drains in more detail later in this section.

The preoperative visit is an exciting time for patients, and they often have many questions as their surgery day draws nearer. This is perfectly normal, so don't feel shy about asking as many questions as you need to ask to feel comfortable about your upcoming procedure.

PERSONAL LIFE CONSIDERATIONS

Preparing for surgery also means making preparations at home and at work. You want to make sure that you get plenty of rest and relaxation while recovering so you can achieve optimal results. But your situation can be less than optimal if your house becomes chaotic from lack of planning, or if you're stressing out because you didn't do enough to cover your responsibilities at work. This is why it's important for you to get your home, your job, your schedule, and your family situated for your recovery.

You're going to need some time off from work to recover, and you'll recover better if you're not stressing out about what's going on at work without you. Talk with your manager and your colleagues about covering for you while you're away. Make sure that someone is handling your duties and keeping in contact with your clients so that you won't be tempted to start working from your recovery bed. Also, discuss the possibility of being away longer than you anticipate should complications arise. It's hard to prepare for that, but complications happen sometimes. In general, knowing that your work is covered and they're prepared for your absence can take a lot of stress off you.

Most of the preparations that moms need to make concern their little ones, and who will help care for them. I discussed this before, because a great source of stress (and sometimes guilt) for moms who are having surgery involves who's caring for the kids. You know that you'll have to take extra care to avoid putting stress on your incisions, and that means taking a break from some of your normal parenting duties, like lifting or carrying small children. Have your spouse, another family member, or a trusted sitter take over as the primary caregiver while you recover.

Here are a few more things that you should think about before surgery and prepare to cover during your downtime:

- **Driving.** You'll need a family member or friend to drive you to and from surgery, but also to possibly be on call to drive you while you recover, because you might be taking pain medication and shouldn't be driving. You could also use car services, and if you haven't used them before, get their apps and learn about them beforehand, so it's one less thing you need to do as your surgery day get closer. But you will not be able to take a car service home from the surgery center. All centers require the name and number of the person responsible to pick you up and bring you home, unless you are headed to the recovery center.

- **A "sitter" for you.** Most patients like to have someone keep tabs on them for the first few days. You are required to have someone stay with you for the first twenty-four hours after a general anesthesia. This person can be especially helpful in the first twenty-four to forty-eight hours as the effects of anesthesia gradually wear off. During this time, you might need help getting up to use the bathroom or to walk around like your surgeon will want you to do to avoid blood clots.

- **Housekeeping help.** You won't be able to do most (if any) housework while your incisions heal, so help with household tasks during recovery will be important. Friends and family can help, but some things can be farmed out, so to speak—for example, use a laundry service, or order groceries online and have them delivered.

- **Pet care.** If you're typically the primary caregiver for the family pets, someone needs to take over the duties of walking the dog and feeding. Older children can pitch in by doing these things for you.

The next sections cover common topics and issues that you and your surgeon will discuss during these pre-op weeks.

MEDICAL HISTORY AND CURRENT MEDICAL PROBLEMS

One of the keys to a safe, successful surgery is to make sure your physician knows everything about your medical history, including any current medical problems. This is a big part of your consultation discussions. But it's also an important part of your pre-op appointment. Even if you already discussed your medical history with your doctor or his staff, don't be surprised if they ask questions about it again, and again, and even again. It's that important.

All surgery comes with risks, but surgeons can minimize risks if they understand any medical issues you have. Chronic conditions can be challenging—like high blood pressure, which can lead to excessive bleeding if the condition isn't well controlled. Diabetes is another disease that raises surgical risks. In this case, the risk of infection after surgery increases. Your surgeon needs to discuss obesity, allergies to medications, blood-clotting problems, and many other conditions that need consideration when developing a surgical plan. It's important to be completely honest and not hold anything back—nothing!—and make sure the surgeon knows about all your medical conditions.

Don't be afraid that having a medical problem will keep you from having the surgery you want. Most medical conditions, even major ones, don't automatically exclude you from having surgery. Generally, your surgeon will want to get medical clearance from your primary care physician. This means he or she consults with your primary doctor to make sure that any conditions you have are well controlled. For some conditions, such as a seizure disorder, the surgeon would likely want to consult any specialists you see regularly, like a neurologist. It's a team approach. Even if you are "cleared" for surgery, the surgeon may decide that it still is not safe for you to proceed. This is up to the surgeon's judgement, because ultimately, he or she is responsible regardless of what physician states you are cleared for surgery.

I recently had to turn down a patient for a breast reconstruction because she had a blood-clotting disorder. Her hematologist would now allow her to stop her blood thinner longer than one day after surgery. The surgery she was going to have was too high risk for bleeding, and together we decided the risk of throwing a blood clot to her lungs was not worth the reward of a possible reconstruction.

Let's say a patient with high blood pressure or diabetes comes to me for surgery. I don't just say, "Hey, you have high blood pressure. You can't have surgery," or, "You have diabetes. It's not safe for you to have surgery." I send them to their primary-care physician for a workup—maybe some lab work or an EKG—so that I can evaluate that patient's surgical risks properly. I'll get the results back, the primary-care physician will make comments about how comfortable and how high or low a risk they think the patient will be, and then I'll assimilate that information. Let's say the doctor thinks the patient is a moderate risk for surgery. After I evaluate everything, I might say to the patient, "Your blood pressure is well controlled. You're a moderate risk. Outside of what your primary-care physician is telling us, I think it's safe to proceed. That doesn't mean surgery isn't risk-free. It means you have a moderate risk." Or I might end up telling the patient that I believe they're at high risk for the procedure we want to do.

Unfortunately, I've turned people away who are a high risk for surgery, and if your risks are high, your surgeon might turn you away, too. Wanting a procedure doesn't equal having it, but it's rare that I have to turn a patient away because of medical problems. Sometimes these things are just out of your control, and your physician might cancel your surgery at the last minute. You might come down with a bad cold or the flu right before your surgery, and if that happens, you'll have to postpone the procedure. I canceled someone's surgery for this very reason because being sick increased her risks, but I was able to perform her surgery safely once she was healthy and recovered.

Consulting with your regular physicians and specialists about any conditions you have is how we surgeons dot our i's and cross our t's to make sure that we're doing the right thing for an elective operation.

MEDICATIONS AND SUPPLEMENTS BEFORE SURGERY

This topic relates closely to your medical history and conditions. Medications and supplements, even in small doses, can have a crucial role in how well your body responds to the surgery. During surgery, specific medicines might be used to help keep blood flowing and the heart pumping, but these medications don't always mix well with prescriptions the patient takes regularly. In some cases, the combination of drugs can lead to serious issues. Once again, you don't want to hold anything back from the surgeon when asked about the medications and supplements you take. If you're not forthcoming, you run the risk of complications during surgery. These complications might be small and uneventful, but every complication is a setback from the overall goal of the surgery. If a surgeon must stop an operation to deal with medication issues, the surgery might not be successfully completed.

Some prescription drugs might have no bearing whatsoever on the actual surgery, but they could lead to issues in the recovery process. For example, if a patient regularly uses opioid or narcotic medication to control pain before a surgery, it will make it much more difficult to control pain after surgery. The best thing to do is consult with your doctor to develop a plan to help decrease or stop your opioid medication before surgery.

In my practice, I strongly urge our patients to avoid certain medications before surgery. I give them a list of prescription and nonprescription products to avoid. Your surgeon will discuss this subject with you in detail during your preoperative visit and will probably give you a similar list. You also should bring a complete list of all the medications you take. For our purposes here, the following general, top-level list gives you an idea of what you'll have to stop taking before surgery:

- **Aspirin or medications that contain aspirin or certain other compounds:** These can cause bleeding problems in normal individuals when taken before or after a surgical procedure, which would make it more difficult for even small incisions to heal. Any other blood thinners or anticoagulants would have the same effect, and you should avoid them for at least two weeks before and after surgery.

- **Oral contraceptive pills and hormone replacement:** Avoid these *if* you have a history of deep vein thrombosis. They increase the risk of forming blood clots. If you don't have this problem, you can likely continue taking these medications, but follow your surgeon's instructions.

- **Diet pills:** Some diet pills can cause heart-rhythm problems when used at the same time as general anesthesia. This is a very simple problem to avoid.

- **Energy drinks:** These aren't medication, but they can interfere with some procedures. Experience has shown that some of the ingredients in such drinks (particularly guarana and high levels of caffeine) can cause heart-rhythm problems when combined with general anesthesia. These ingredients on their own can cause high blood pressure and heart palpitations.

- **Supplements:** Just because supplements aren't technically medication doesn't mean they can't put patients at risk during surgery, too. Gingko biloba, ginseng, and fish oil can increase the risk of bleeding. Garlic and ephedra have been associated with cardiovascular risk. Other supplements can increase the skin's sensitivity to light, which can complicate laser skin treatments.

PRESURGERY SHOPPING LIST

Your presurgical preparations include shopping for items you'll need before and after surgery. Your doctor will give you a list of things you'll need; this will include general items (some for your comfort during recovery) as well as items that are specific to your type of surgery. It's best to go shopping as soon as you get the list to make sure you have what you'll need after surgery and to take pressure off of yourself in the final days before your procedure. The last thing you need to do then is go running all over town trying to gather the items on the list.

I like my patients to get the following items before their surgery. No matter the procedure, these will help you during recovery:

- **Water or clear soda (not diet):** ginger ale or lemon-lime soda, for example

- **Plain crackers:** saltines or toast

- **Soup:** clear broths that aren't cream based

- **Gelatin dessert:** like Jell-O, but not the diet variety

- **Fruit purée:** applesauce or any similar kind

- **Prescriptions:** all prescription and over-the-counter medications the surgeon wants you to have after the procedure

- **Arnica montana:** an herbal supplement to prevent bruising and swelling

- **Hibiclens:** a presurgery cleanser to use in the shower the night before and the morning of surgery

- **Antibiotic ointment:** Bacitracin and Polysporin, but *never Neosporin (Some people can have an allergic reaction to this product, and it's known to cause allergic reactions in wounds, so I avoid it.)*

- **Hydrogen peroxide:** can be mixed with sterile water to clean and remove dried blood and scabs where needed, but don't use for routine wound cleaning (it can impede normal healing)

- **Underwear liners:** to use on scars like a wound pad because they're clean and absorbent

- **Gauze pads (4" x 4") and paper tape:** for dressing changes for many of the surgeries, though not all.

Many patients think that sports drinks will help keep them hydrated. I'm personally against these drinks because of their high sugar content. It's best to stick with water and clear soda, preferably sugar free.

CLEANSING BEFORE SURGERY

I included the presurgery cleanser Hibiclens in the shopping list, so I want to explain more about why you need this and how to use it. Everyone has germs or bacteria on their skin that can potentially cause surgical-wound infections. To reduce germs on your skin before surgery, you should bathe or shower with a mild soap or, preferably, an antiseptic skin cleanser with chlorhexidine that kills bacteria. (You can find such products at most pharmacies.) I give my patients Hibiclens, which can continue killing pathogens for up to twenty-four hours, and repeated use has a cumulative effect. This is why all surgery centers and most surgeons ask patients to use it the night before and the morning of surgery.

Shower the night before and the morning of your surgery, using Hibiclens the same way you'd use soap. However, Hibiclens is toxic to mucus membranes, so avoid getting it in your ears, eyes, nose, mouth, open wounds, or in the genital area. First, wash your face and hair with whatever shampoo you'd normally use, then finish washing your body with Hibiclens. You'll notice that it doesn't lather, unlike your regular shampoo or soap. For best results, do the following:

- Thoroughly rinse your skin with water.

- Apply Hibiclens or similar soap to your washcloth, and wash your entire body gently, especially the surgical-site area.

- Rinse thoroughly.

- Don't use lotions, powders, or deodorants after washing, because many have chemicals that interfere with the cleanser's bacteria-killing action.

- Don't shave any body hair in the planned surgical site.

THE DAY BEFORE SURGERY

You're almost there! The day before surgery is often exciting for patients. There are a few important things that need to be done, and I emphasize the following to my patients so that they're absolutely ready on the day of surgery:

- Confirm your surgery time with your physician's office. This is important, because sometimes schedules have to change, and you want to arrive for surgery at the right time. You might take a practice run to the surgery center so that you know where you're going and won't be late.

- Be sure you've filled any prescriptions ahead of time, so you don't have to stop for them on the way home from surgery. Set out your medications and your medication-tracking log (provided at your consultation) where you can find them easily when you get home.

- Cleanse the surgical areas the night before surgery. Take a shower the night before and wash the surgical areas with mild soap, but don't shave any hair the night before. Use any surgical soap your surgeon might have given to you such as Hibiclens.

- Don't eat or drink anything after midnight the night before surgery. This includes water.

REPEAT: DON'T EAT OR DRINK ANYTHING AFTER MIDNIGHT

I can't stress this enough: don't eat *anything* after midnight before your surgery. This is so important, and yet people will often try to sneak in a snack after the time their doctor told them to stop all food and drink. Don't do it! Your stomach has to be empty before going under general anesthesia. Why? General anesthesia relaxes your digestive-tract muscles and airway that keeps food and stomach acid from going from your stomach into your lungs. With those reflexes essentially stopped, there's a risk of vomiting or regurgitating and aspirating the contents, which can cause damage to the lungs, or worse. I usually tell patients that they can't eat or drink after midnight before surgery. It's also important to avoid alcohol—especially red wine—for a few days before surgery, because it thins the blood.

However, don't stop taking any prescription medications unless your surgeon instructs you to do so. If you normally take a blood pressure pill or thyroid pill in the morning, for example, you can take the pill with a small sip of water. It's important to keep taking that kind of medication at the same time of day to control any medical conditions.

In the next chapter, I'll describe what you can expect on the day of your surgery.

CHAPTER 12

The Day of Surgery

Your surgery day has arrived! Many things that happen on the day of surgery are specific to the procedure, but in this chapter, I'm going to walk you through the general aspects of a typical surgery day so you can get some insight into the surgery experience from start to finish. Let's go!

THE MORNING OF SURGERY

You'll wake up excited and anticipating your transformation. Here are some important things you need to do before you go to the surgery center:

- Don't eat or drink anything! I can't repeat this enough. Take any daily prescription medication that you must have with a sip of water in the early morning.

- Brush your teeth the morning of surgery, but don't swallow any gulps of water.

- Shower and wash the surgical areas again with mild soap or the soap your surgeon gave you, but don't shave any hair.

- Don't wear moisturizers, creams, lotions, or makeup of any kind.

- Wear only comfortable, loose-fitting clothing that doesn't go over your head. Remove hairpins, wigs, piercings, and jewelry. Leave all valuables at home.

- Report to the surgery center or hospital one to two hours before your scheduled surgery. Call the facility for its specific rules about when to arrive. A parent or legal guardian must accompany patients under age eighteen.

A TYPICAL SURGERY DAY

You might feel a little nervous when you wake up on the day of surgery. Some patients are nervous and excited, some are a bit scared—maybe they're scared of getting an IV, even though they discussed it at length with their surgeons. My best advice is to relax and remember how much you've been looking forward to your surgery. Remember these three things:

1. **Trust your surgeon.** You did your research and made an excellent choice!

2. **Trust yourself.** You made a highly informed choice to have your surgery, and it's something you want.

3. **Stay off the Internet.** Avoid reading what others say on the Internet—again, all patients are different and have different experiences. Trust what your doctor tells you.

Generally, the surgical facility will expect you to be there one to two hours ahead of your scheduled surgery time. If the surgeon has several cases scheduled that day and you're not the first case of the day, be prepared for delays and possibly not going into surgery exactly at your scheduled time.

The surgery-center staff will greet you when you arrive. Don't be surprised or annoyed, but they'll take your medical history yet again. Many different people might ask you the same questions repeatedly at this time because they're trying at many different levels to make sure that no one misses anything in your medical history. For example, four different people might ask you if you're allergic to any medications. They're just triple-checking themselves, and everyone has a job to do, so expect to repeat your health history a few times. Just relax and appreciate the extra care that everyone's taking to make sure your surgery proceeds smoothly and safely.

Next, the staff will take you to the preoperative area where you'll change into a surgical gown and put all of your personal belongings into a bag. You might be able to visit with your spouse or partner at this time, depending on the facility's rules. But you can usually see your support person after you're in your gown and in a bed.

You might need to take care of some paperwork before you get your IV—again depending on the facility. I like to take care of everything before the surgery day, but some places still need you to sign documents or deal with some financial aspects that day at the surgery center. The staff might ask you some questions about financial matters.

Now it's really time to get going. The pre-op nurses will place an IV into your arm. The anesthesiologist will give you the anesthesia that puts you to sleep through this IV, but the nurses will give you fluids first. Your surgery is about an hour away at this point. After the

IV is in place, the anesthesiologist will come in and explain which drugs will be used—and why they'll be used—and answer any final questions you might have about the anesthesia. You'll also sign an informed consent for anesthesia. Next, the surgeon will come in to talk with you, make sure you're doing okay, and generally make some small talk to help you relax. The surgeon might also review a few final details of your procedure. Such as confirming the implant size for a breast implant, or marking the areas to be treated. for liposuction. In fact, the surgeon will usually make surgical markings for any procedures that need them at this time. After the surgical markings, you can ask any final questions you might have.

Your support person can usually stay with you until the anesthesiologist comes to take you to the operating room. You usually get some kind of an antianxiety medication before going to the operating room just to take the edge off, particularly if you're a bit nervous. Your support person can either wait for you or leave and come back, depending on the procedure. If it's a six- or seven-hour procedure, your surgeon will probably want to come back and see you when you're in recovery. The staff will give your support person instructions, and that person should their leave contact information with the staff.

The anesthesiologist and the nurse will accompany you to the operating room, and staff will wheel you in on a patient cart. Be prepared to see a cold, more sterile environment in the operating room. It's usually kept cold to decrease infection risk. You might meet more staff in the operating room, like the scrub technician who helps the surgeon during surgery or any other nursing staff who might be in the room helping with the case. The staff wheels the patient cart next to the operating room bed, and will ask you to slide over to the operating bed, usually under your own power. It's a narrow bed, but the staff will guide you and get you in the right position, even if you feel woozy from the relaxation medication.

At this point, you'll probably hear some strange mechanical noises coming from the anesthesia machine. You'll also hear the sounds of people in the room moving equipment around and getting set up. Hopefully, none of this will make you nervous, and it shouldn't. Just expect a little bit of organized chaos to be going on in the room. You'll probably be feeling fairly relaxed at this point anyway, thanks to the antianxiety medication. The staff will cover you with a warm blanket and put compression stockings or sleeves on your legs to prevent blood clotting. The nurses will connect you to monitors to manage your vital signs before the anesthesiology team takes over and puts you to sleep.

The nurses will take your vital signs before you go under anesthesia to make sure your blood pressure is okay. They'll make sure you're comfortable, and then put the oxygen mask on your face so you can breathe some oxygen before you get anything in the IV that's going to put you to sleep. Then the anesthesia staff will talk you through the next steps. They'll give you the anesthesia medication through your IV—and you might feel some burning in the IV when the medication goes in. Anesthesia staff will often give patients something before that to numb the blood vessels, but it doesn't always work, so you still might feel a little bit of burning. And then you'll just drift off to sleep. Have a good dream, and we'll see you in recovery!

After you go to sleep, that's it—you generally won't remember anything else until you've been in recovery for about an hour. You might not even remember going into the operating room because of the relaxing antianxiety medication you had earlier. The first thing you might feel when you wake up might not be pain, but rather disorientation. You might literally wonder, "Where am I? What's going on? Are we done?" Everyone wakes up from anesthesia differently, but usually patients are in recovery for at least an hour before they wake up fully. To show just how disoriented anesthesia can make you, I'll tell you about the most common thing that happens with patients in post-op. Sometimes they'll say something like, "The nursing staff rushed me out of post-op. I wasn't there very long." They don't realize that they've been in recovery for an hour but awake for only five or ten minutes, so they feel like the staff rushed them out. The staff moves you out as soon as you're awake, because another patient will be coming out of the operating room soon. The staff is never rushing patients out of the recovery center. The patients don't have any concept of time at this point, and they don't realize how long they've been there.

If you're not staying overnight, your support person will come into the recovery room to greet you. The staff will remove your IV and help you get into your clothes. You'll leave the facility in a wheelchair, even if you could walk out under your own power. Staff will help you get into your vehicle, and you can go home. If you're going to a recovery center instead of home, medical-transportation staff will take you there. Patients are sometimes so out of it from the anesthesia that they might not even remember the trip to the recovery center, and the first time they might be awake is when the recovery center staff wakes them. Personally, I often operate at a hospital that has a recovery center, so that patients don't need to leave the facility to go to recovery.

What I just described is a typical surgery-day experience, and this experience is generally what you can expect. When you get home, you'll start your recovery process, and I talk about that in the next chapter.

One more thing: Many of my patients come from out of town to my office in Arizona. Those patients need to stay in town for at least one week after surgery, possibly two weeks. Out-of-towners might spend the first night at a recovery center and the rest of their stay in a hotel, if they don't have friends or family in town. If they're alone in town and don't have anyone to help them, my office can arrange for care during the recovery process at extra expense to the patient.

ABOUT ANESTHESIA

If you've never been under general anesthesia before, you might be a little nervous about it. But I want to put your mind at ease, because I was nervous about it the first time I had surgery, too. I was scared to go to sleep, thinking about what my family and kids would do if something happened to me—and I knew all about how safe anesthesia is and had plenty of colleagues who reinforced and validated what I knew. Still, I had the jitters—and it's normal to feel that way. Anesthesia is quite safe when administered correctly by trained anesthesiologists. So, what's the source of these jittery feelings?

I think that the media drives a lot of that fear, and patients probably see or hear stories about people who had serious complications or even died from anesthesia. It happens, but you have to dig deeper into those stories to find out why those things occurred. Many times, it's because the people who administered the anesthesia weren't fully trained to do so, or they erred in evaluating the individual patient's safety based on medical history. Unfortunately, these stories are often about someone undergoing a cosmetic-surgery procedure—which makes matters worse for businesses like mine— but again, you need to look at what was really going on. Was the surgeon board-certified in plastic surgery? Maybe not, and a lot of people who die in those situations might not have done their research and made a poor choice of surgeon. Media outlets report and sensationalize these stories without realizing that the surgeon involved isn't the average, skilled, safe surgeon. You're hearing only about the few times a year that something goes horribly wrong, and you're not hearing about the thousands of safe, successful surgeries performed every year. You're also not hearing about the patients' problems—they might have had medical issues that led to complications and created the situation, like a cardiac problem.

The fact is that most of us board-certified plastic surgeons will never experience serious anesthesia-related complications or death in a healthy patient in our entire careers. If it does ever happen, it's usually an unforeseen cardiac abnormality or some other condition that we would have never known about. Again, it's so rare for that to happen. At the risk of sounding cliché, you're more likely to die in a car accident on the way to the doctor's office than you are from being under anesthesia. Unless the surgeon is performing an operation that he shouldn't be performing because a patient has chronic diseases or conditions, everything will be fine. If you received preoperative clearance and your surgeon evaluated your risks *and* you're at the point where you're having surgery, anything that might happen to you from this point forward would be the rarest, unluckiest thing—or the surgeon wouldn't be operating on you in the first place.

I want to mention possible side effects. Everyone handles anesthesia differently. One patient might go to sleep, wake up, and feel fine, though drowsy. Another patient might have nausea and vomiting the first twenty-four to forty-eight hours after surgery, and that's normal, too. Either way, when facing surgery, you should prepare for the possibility of such side effects.

BE PATIENT

You'll probably be excited when the surgery is over and want to look at the results right away. It's important to be patient and not remove any special postsurgery garments until your physician tells you that it's okay to do so. Your doctor might see you the next day or sometimes not for a few days after surgery, but when you do see him, you'll find out when you can take your garments off. Being patient can help your recovery go quickly and smoothly, so read on to learn more about what happens after your surgery.

CHAPTER 13

What to Expect after Surgery

Your focus after surgery should be on healing as quickly and as effectively as possible. That means you should take responsibility for your own recovery by following your doctor's advice to ensure a smooth healing process and lasting results. The next sections give you a lot of information to help you kick off a great recovery process, including simple tips to follow that I know have helped my own patients relax, heal well, and have great outcomes.

YOUR POSTOPERATIVE APPOINTMENTS

After your surgery, you can ensure the best opportunity for healing by getting enough rest, hydrating, taking your medications as prescribed, and avoiding exercise or strenuous activity. Another important step in your healing process is to make sure you keep all your postoperative appointments with your surgeon or his staff. Generally, your postoperative appointments let your surgeon take a closer look to make sure that you're healing properly. But it's also a way for you and your physician to keep tabs on your recovery plan and make sure you're correctly following the plan and all of the instructions that your doctor gave you before surgery. I like to schedule my patients' postoperative appointments before their surgery, and these appointments are part of the overall recovery process. Your first postsurgery appointment should take place in one to seven days after your surgery. During the appointments, I monitor how the incisions are healing and assess bruising and swelling, overall pain or discomfort, and how well patients are adhering to their recovery plans. I also evaluate the medication record and surgical drains, if they're involved.

Don't be tempted to skip any of your postoperative appointments. I know that it sometimes feels inconvenient to make time to go to these appointments when patients get back into their normal routines. But these appointments are a crucial part of the long recovery process. They're important for your own peace of mind, because you know that there's a specific plan in place for monitoring and tracking your recovery from surgery. For me, staying in close contact with each patient throughout the entire recovery process is a top priority.

RIGHT AFTER SURGERY

As I stated, the most important thing to do right after surgery is to keep that first postoperative appointment, because this is when your surgeon starts to monitor your healing. The next sections describe how you can expect the healing process to proceed.

BRUISING AND SWELLING

Bruising and swelling are par for the course with plastic surgery, and I discussed both in the procedures sections. But seeing the bruises and swelling right after surgery and for a few days beyond can be a bit disheartening or at least concerning. Regardless of the procedure, you'll have some kind of bruising and swelling, and it's completely normal. Even if your plastic surgeon is gentle, chances are you'll still have some bruising, simply because surgery is traumatic and causes some bleeding beneath the skin. When we operate, we're creating a controlled, large wound. Blood cells settle beneath the skin and go through the natural changes of any bruise, causing the skin to look black and blue and eventually a yellow color before returning to normal—these are the stages of bruise healing. Little capillaries also break, and you bleed in your skin. You might notice that the bruised area isn't tender. The collection of blood cells makes it look worse than it is.

Some procedures cause more bruising than others. Liposuction, for example, can result in a lot of bruising and is probably the worst, because moving the suction instrument around under the skin causes a lot of trauma. You don't see that much bruising with breast surgery, but it happens. Facial procedures tend to bruise a lot, and that can really cause patients anxiety. But no matter where the bruises are, don't worry; they'll start to fade soon after surgery. Taking arnica montana and bromelain supplements can help reduce bruising and swelling, and you should discuss these supplements with your surgeon.

INCISIONS AND SCARS

Your incisions need care to make sure they heal well and minimize scarring as much as possible. There's no way around it: incisions look awful right after surgery, and they can leak fluid that often worries patients, particularly when they take a bandage off and see the fluids on it. This is completely normal. Sometimes, fluid leakage can occur for several weeks, or maybe only a little bit of fluid will weep out of the incisions. If you're having a liposuction procedure, be prepared to see a lot of fluid leakage, because the surgeon injects a lot of liquid during the procedure, and some of it seeps out afterward.

The incision's appearance is the other thing that concerns patients and often makes them feel a little panicky. Suturing the skin can make the incision look and feel lumpy, bumpy, and firm. It's not a nice, smooth scar right away; that usually takes two to three months to happen. Dissolvable stitches will disappear after about two months, and that's when scars start to flatten out—the stitches being what gave the incision a bad appearance. Surgeons suture the incision in a specific way to alleviate tension on the scar—because tension is one of the things that leads to a poor scar. The suture that's making the incision look bad right after surgery is actually going to prevent it from looking bad permanently.

It can take a year for scars to mature. They take time to become what they're going to be and will change continuously for the better over the months. Scars are reddish in color for a long time, because they have a robust blood supply to enable them to produce the collagen that fills a scar. As that process approaches one year, scars start to fade back to a lighter color that looks more like your normal skin tone. I try to educate patients, so they understand that scars change so much from six weeks to one year. So, when I say, "Be patient," I really mean it. Here's the scarring process in a nutshell:

- **The first six weeks:** Things will look the worst during this time—inflamed and swollen with lumpy, bumpy scars.

- **Two to three months:** You should see lots of improvement in the appearance of scars. They tend to improve greatly during this time.

- **Four, five, and six months:** You should see even more improvement, and that will make you feel great.

- **One year:** Your scars should be matured and doing great at this point.

WASH AFTER SURGERY

I mentioned showering or bathing with Hibiclens before surgery. After surgery, you'll use a regular antibacterial soap instead of Hibiclens. You need to take showers after surgery, not baths, for about three to four weeks because you can't soak your incisions until completely closed.

I give my patients a lot of tips and advice right after surgery to help them have the best recovery possible. The next sections cover some of the things I tell my patients to do in the weeks and months after surgery.

LISTEN TO YOUR DOCTOR'S ADVICE

This is the most important piece of advice I can give you, above all else. Your doctor will provide you with general and procedure-specific recovery advice that you should follow to the letter. A common mistake that many patients make after plastic surgery is not following their doctor's orders as closely as they should. Having a good day or two doesn't mean you should start feeling that the worst is behind you and that some of the stricter orders no longer apply. It's extremely important to continue following your doctor's instructions throughout the recovery time. This includes diet suggestions, applying ice (or not applying it), and taking any medications. Your ability to follow the doctor's advice can definitely speed up the recovery time.

RELAX

It's highly important for you to take time off from your everyday activities to just relax and heal. Don't fool yourself into thinking that you can jump right back into your normal routine immediately when you first get home. Know and understand the limitations that will prevent you from doing even some of the most mundane and simple tasks. Make a list of the daily tasks that you would normally do, and then honestly determine which of those tasks you'll be able to handle. Overexerting yourself will only delay your recovery. Even if you're feeling great, don't jump up and start doing your normal activities, because you could damage incisions and reopen wounds, or worse. Chill and enjoy your time off. Mommies—and everyone these days—are doers and goers, and it seems that patients can't really wrap their heads around just being calm and not doing too much. It makes such a big difference when patients don't listen to their doctors and are too overactive or try to get back to what's normal too quickly. Then they're in pain, and things don't feel right.

RELY ON OTHERS

This one goes with the previous tip. It's easy to let yourself believe that because your plastic surgery was elective, you shouldn't be entitled to the same care and support from others that you would want if it were a nonelective surgery. Get past this line of thinking right away. The truth is, you'll definitely need the help and support of loved ones and friends to help you get through this. Make sure you're okay with relying on others, whether it's accepting help from a friend or family member to take your kids to and from school or letting someone help you go to and from the bathroom for the first two or so days.

AVOID TOO MUCH SUN

You must avoid sun exposure to your scars for up to one year. Too much sun on young scars can lead to darkened scars (hyperpigmentation.) Too much heat may lead to increased swelling in young wounds and surgical sites and should be avoided for the first week at the very least. When you do go out again, be sure to cover your incision sites with clothing, wear hats or visors, and use sunscreen. Sunscreen should not be used on the incisions themselves, however, until directed by your surgeon.

DRINK PLENTY OF WATER

Staying fully hydrated after surgery is crucial for recovery. Water is a great catalyst to your recovery, and it helps your body get rid of toxins from the anesthesia. Be sure you have water on hand at all times to keep yourself hydrated. Water helps keep things in balance and ensures that your surgery heals quickly and effectively. I prefer water to any sports drink or soda any day. Eating well is also important—so important that I'll get into more detail on it in the next section.

AVOID STRENUOUS EXERCISE

This should be a no-brainer because you have incisions that can open from stretching and pulling on them. Also, increasing your heart rate increases the risk of bleeding. If you're used to a vigorous workout routine, you'll have to ease back into it slowly and avoid any strenuous exercise for about four to six weeks. Be sure to discuss your usual workout routine with your doctor so you can both plan for when and how you'll get back to your normal exercise regimen again. You should do nothing until your doctor tells you that you can. In general, you shouldn't do anything strenuous for six weeks. I sometimes allow my patients to restart cardiac-related activity at four weeks, but most surgeons won't fully release a patient for six weeks. It won't be as hard to do as it sounds—you'll be sore for the first two to three weeks and won't want to do anything, and the last two to three weeks go by so quickly that you'll hardly notice.

... BUT DON'T BE STATIONARY

Lying around after surgery can lead to blood clots, so you need to get up and move. I like to get my patients up and moving while wearing their compression stockings on day one. I know the anesthesia will make them feel sluggish when they get home after surgery. But walking to the bathroom and taking a short stroll in the house every hour (like walking to the kitchen and back) can help you avoid lung infections, pneumonia, and blood clots that can come from lying in bed or sitting in a chair all day.

I give my patients activity timelines that are time-tested, so we know how long you should take to recover. You need to give your body the chance to heal. Surgeons want you to have the best outcome and a smooth recovery, and we don't want you to compromise your results by doing something too quickly. So, don't go picking the babies up out of the crib after a breast augmentation—because you can undo a great procedure that way.

ABOUT YOUR MEDICATIONS

Your physician typically gives you four medications: a pain pill, an antibiotic, an anti-nausea pill, and an antianxiety pill that helps relax muscle spasms. It's best to try to settle your stomach before you start taking your medication. Start with sips of a water on your way home from the surgery center. Sometimes drinks like clear soda help settle the stomach, but they should not become routine. Try the following steps for taking your pain medication:

- Slowly advance your liquid intake and eat some crackers when you're able, then take your first pain pill when your stomach feels more settled.

- Keep eating and drinking, then continue taking your pills according to your surgeon's directions.

- Go back to sipping liquids if the pills are upsetting your stomach.

- Stop the narcotic pain medicine as soon as you can, but do not be afraid to use them when needed. If your physician approves, it might be okay to take Tylenol only or Ibuprofen. Your physician should give you instructions as to how much and how often to take them. Typical over-the-counter narcotics have Tylenol in them as well. An overdose of Tylenol can harm the liver, so you must keep meticulous record of how much Tylenol you take in a twenty-four-hour period, and never exceed recommended doses found on the side of the bottle.

Your surgeon will give you an antibiotic through your IV on the morning of surgery. This lasts for about eight hours, depending on the type of antibiotic, so take your first antibiotic pill when your physician tells you to, then continue taking it according to the directions on your prescription until they're gone. You should take the anti-nausea pill and the antianxiety pill as needed. Patients often use the antianxiety pills to help them sleep, because they can be more effective than the pain medication.

MORE ABOUT SURGICAL DRAINS

The need for surgical drains depends on the procedure and relates to the area of the body and how much tissue the surgeon has to elevate. But if you do need drains, you'll have to take proper care of them after surgery because they perform an important function in your healing process.

A tummy-tuck procedure, for example, requires drains in most cases. The surgeon makes an incision across the lower part of the abdomen and the pubic region, and then elevates the skin all the way up to the rib cage. When you lift the skin off the underlying muscles, you can't just lay it back down and not expect any fluid to collect in that space, as with any external wound. Separating the skin from the muscles is an internal wound. If the surgeon lays the skin back down on top of the muscle without placing a drain in there, a lot of fluid would collect under the skin and cause a postoperative seroma—a fluid-filled bump. In the tummy-tuck area, a seroma could get so big that the patient might look pregnant! The fluid in small seromas would eventually absorb into the body, but they also prevent normal healing and affect the overall cosmetic contour. Physicians will drain large seromas in the office, and they might need to replace any drain that they removed.

Drains prevent seromas by directing fluid out of the body and away from the incision site until the body can reabsorb the remaining fluid on its own through the lymphatic system, which is the system that runs throughout the body and helps drain any liquid that collects in our tissue. Our lymphatics drain through the lymphatic channels back to lymph nodes every day, all the time. In a procedure like a tummy tuck, the surgeon disrupts the connections of some of those lymphatics. It can take two to three months for lymphatics to completely regain their function and this is why swelling lasts two to three months. The drain is in place to allow the overlying skin to scar down to the underlying structures which obliterates the space and deters the formation of seroma fluid collections. However, the drain is usually needed for only seven to ten days. Once the skin is adequately scarred down, the drain is removed.

Any procedure that doesn't create a big space won't need drains. I don't usually need to use drains when I perform an arm lift, for example, because I close down the entire space when I close the arms. I also don't use them in most breast reductions or an augmentation, because the implant fills the space.

As I mentioned, patients need drains for about seven to ten days, but sometimes they need them longer, and surgeons determine that by how much fluid they're putting out. It's safe to remove the drains when there's very little fluid collection, because that means the space has healed enough and the lymphatics can start doing their job again. The surgeon will leave drains in place if they're still putting out more fluid than he or she would like to see.

WHAT "HEALED" MEANS

The hardest part of describing postsurgery recovery is defining what "healed" means to an individual patient, because all patients are different and will recover differently and at different rates. Achieving the final results happens in stages. But because recovery from different procedures is also different, it's impossible to state with absolute certainty that any patient will recover fully by a specific time. This is why it's important to talk with your surgeon in detail about your expectations for healing results, and you should spend time in your consultation on this subject so that you can fully understand what to expect.

IF SURGERY DOESN'T MEET YOUR EXPECTATIONS

I've already discussed managing a patient's expectations before surgery so that there are no surprises or disappointments after surgery. But despite any surgeon's best efforts to manage expectations, some patients can't let go of what they wanted their breasts to look like, how flat they wanted their tummy to be, how much more lifted they wanted their thighs, or how much smaller they wanted their arms. As a surgeon, I can try to paint a realistic picture for the patient, but sometimes a patient subconsciously ignores what I say as not realistic, and in the end, expects a result that isn't possible, and that is frustrating for the patient and for me. When talking with patients about expectations, I ask them to do some soul searching on our presurgery discussions about what's realistic and what's not. I ask them to not be disappointed if that perfect result that's in their mind didn't happen or if a scar is a bit crooked in one spot compared with another spot, and so on. As surgeons, we do everything we can to make things as perfectly symmetric as possible, but because natural asymmetries can become more enhanced in some cases (breast augmentation, for example), you just can't always achieve perfect symmetry, despite us chasing it. Early, during healing, patients can become frustrated, but I tell them that it's early and they need to understand that it takes time to start seeing certain improvements. I know it can be hard not to be concerned, but patients need to relax for the first two to three months, because so much changes during that time.

Surgeons know that patients can get panicky about certain things. Just be open with your surgeon if you're feeling that the reality doesn't meet your expectations, and he or she will be happy to reassure you. I encourage patients to call me instead of bottling all of that up inside. But if I tell them that they just need to give it time, I don't want them calling my nurse every day to say that it still hasn't gotten better. Part of the problem is that friends tell them how their recoveries should be. But the friend's result and recovery just aren't a good indicator of how everyone else's recovery will progress. I try to bring them back to the reality that everybody is different.

POSTPROCEDURE BLUES

This is a good place to discuss something I call the postprocedure blues. Most women will be really excited about having surgery—they get pumped, they don't care about all of the incisions, and they can't wait to see their final results. But when some women come back for their follow-up visit, I can tell they're just not feeling right and that something's going on in their heads. That "something" is usually the postprocedure blues.

Sometimes postprocedure depression or blues happens when patients are feeling guilty for having a procedure that has them feeling laid up and not able to perform daily duties. These thoughts can creep in during recovery, when patients are resting and have a lot of time to think about what's happened. At this point, patients could be relying heavily on family and friends for their basic needs, which can lead to feelings of frustration and dependency and make matters even worse. They can feel remorse after a procedure and wonder, "Why did I do this to myself?" They might even wonder why they had the surgery in the first place. Such thoughts are fairly common and can come from the patients feeling guilty that maybe having surgery was selfish, so they feel down about themselves. Patients usually lose the blues, though, along with those other negative feelings.

I typically just talk about it with these patients. For example, one patient became depressed when she realized she couldn't pick up her son, Jason, after the surgery, because her doctor restricted her from lifting more than ten to twenty pounds. She had anxiety about it that led to the postprocedure blues, and she questioned why she even had the surgery and had thoughts about being selfish. I told her that although it's true that she couldn't lift her young son, he could crawl up on the couch and get into her lap. She could still snuggle with him and give and get hugs. I also reminded her that because she's a mom, she probably just isn't used to putting herself first and felt guilty because she couldn't do everything she normally did for her family right away after her surgery. Moms need to know that it's okay to put themselves first sometimes, and it's not as if they're changing how they feel about their kids and family by doing that. This particular mom also needed to remember that she went through this surgery for a reason and was trying to get something back into her life that she felt was missing. This all brought her back around to the reality that it was only a matter of time before she could return to her normal routine—including picking Jason up again—and her reward for being patient was her new self.

Final results can take time to achieve. It can sometimes be two to six months before things settle. Some women lose patience while waiting this long and can become discouraged. Patients just need to get past an attitude of wanting immediate results and remember that everything will be back to normal soon. It can be easy to lose sight of the personal satisfaction that your surgery will bring you when you've healed fully. Relax and be patient—the new you is coming.

CHAPTER 14

The New-You Lifestyle—You Can Have Your Cake and Eat It, Too

Your surgery results depend a lot on what you do in the months and years after you finally say goodbye to your surgeon. Maintaining your results means adopting a lifestyle that's healthy and will support lasting results—and your lasting satisfaction. You can do this with healthy eating and regular exercise to maintain the changes your surgery made to your body. If you had a tummy tuck, for example, you simply can't go back to being a junk food junkie. The best tuck in the world won't last if you slouch on the couch and eat cheese puffs and ice cream every night.

The bottom line is this: Having surgery isn't a license to misbehave and go back to old, bad habits. Personally, I work hard at being healthy and fit. I've learned a lot about nutrition and exercise, and you can, too. Educating yourself about nutrition and exercise and putting what you've learned to work is all highly important to maintaining your results and protecting the financial investment you made in yourself. If you had bad habits before surgery, you'll need to develop new, healthier habits before and after surgery. The upside is that if you live a healthy lifestyle 90 percent of the time, you can eat cookies and cake occasionally, and have some chocolate and ice cream as special treats—just don't go overboard—and you can still be thin, fit, and in shape.

You just have to remember one thing: *A successful patient is one who's willing to put in the work to maintain the results.*

How do you do that? Again, everyone is different, and what one person finds satisfying and easy to do and sustain might be really difficult for another person. You need to find a way of eating and staying fit that works for you. I can't tell you to go to the gym three times a week and do cardio six days a week—that might work for me, but it won't necessarily be something that you or anyone else will enjoy and sustain. The same goes for a meal plan—it should be something that you can live with every day. It's taken me years to figure out what works for my body. I function well on a high-fat meal plan. I don't do well with high-carb eating because I get bloaty and gassy. Although high-fat plans work well for me, someone else might do horribly eating the same way and need a higher-carbohydrate or higher-protein way of eating.

Whatever plans you make for eating and exercising for health and fitness, understand that you can't expect to have liposuction and a tummy tuck and continue to eat as much chocolate, sugar, and unhealthy foods as you want all the time. You can't have 1,500 calories of Twinkies every day if you're on a 1,500-calorie meal plan and think that you're going to be healthy. Doing that won't give you a long-lasting result. It's about what you eat, and definitely not only about how much you eat.

You can't simply wish the lifestyle upon yourself—you have to do it. You have to live it and be intentional! And if you want to be happy with all the good money you spent for a good surgeon to do a good operation, you have to help that surgeon help you. That means trying to live between the lines 85 to 90 percent of the time with how you eat and take care of yourself. That applies to smoking, too. One of my favorite motivational speakers, Zig Ziglar, says that if you aim at nothing, you'll hit it every time. It's true, and I like to quote that to my patients who claim that they've done everything they can to lose weight. I know it can be hard, and I'm not making fun of them. I'm just trying to help people understand that they probably haven't done everything they can.

Consider these questions:

- What do you do for exercise?

- How long do you exercise?

- What kinds of foods do you eat?

- Do you track what you actually eat?

- Do you know how many calories you take in each day?

- Do you know about how many calories you burn each day?

If you can answer those questions honestly, you'll know whether you need to do more work on improving your lifestyle so that you can maintain your surgery results. The foundation for all of this is very simple: there's a specific number of calories that you need to take in, and then an amount you need to burn to lose weight—calories in, calories out. You need to burn more calories than you take in if you want to lose weight. If you're not keeping track of what you eat, how much you eat, and the basic content of that food (fat and sugar content, for example), then you don't really know and can't say that you're doing or have done everything you can to lose weight. That's when I can help my patients with suggestions and maybe point them to a nutrition specialist who can teach them how to track what they eat every day. If you need that kind of help, talk with your surgeon or your family physician.

WHAT I DO TO STAY HEALTHY AND FIT

I've mentioned that I'm a healthy and fit kind of guy, and I'm really into it. So, you probably wonder what I do for myself to stay healthy. I can tell you, though what works for me might not be what's best for you. You'll need to find out what works best for your lifestyle. I'm not a nutritionist. I'm just a guy who wants to stay healthy and fit, has done a lot of research, and has learned through trial and error what works best for me. I can tell you about the basic principles I follow, and maybe that will help you get started on your own journey to health. The following are my basic principles for staying healthy and fit—I try to stick with them, and they've served me well:

- **Water:** I try to drink at least a gallon of water a day, if not more. Your body can't perform at its best if you don't stay hydrated.

- **Meals:** I work on having a well-balanced meal plan of carbohydrates, fats, and proteins, and I stick with good fruits, vegetables, and proteins. I follow calorie control and portion control, and I indulge when I can—without going overboard, and that's the important thing. Indulging occasionally can keep you from feeling deprived and really help you stick with your healthy meal plan. Again, just don't overdo it.

- **Sugar:** I stay away from sugar as if it's the devil. I know people are going to eat sugar, and though I feel very strongly about it, even I eat sugar sometimes. But sugar's a problem, and I avoid it as much as I can.

- **Processed foods:** I avoid processed foods as much as possible. My rule of thumb is that if it doesn't have a mother or grow in the ground, it's processed. If it's not salt-of-the-earth proteins, fruits, and vegetables, it's processed. Does that eliminate anything in a package? Not necessarily. If your favorite granola's ingredients list says something like, "oats, raisins, nuts, cinnamon, and coconut flakes," and that's all, the fact that it comes in a package is less important. You should be concerned when you see chemical words that are twenty letters long, and you can't pronounce them.

Those are my principles in a nutshell, and they work quite well for me. Another thing I do is track my calories and macros. Macros are macronutrients, which are carbohydrates, fats, and proteins. It's one thing to track the foods you eat, but you should also know how those foods affect your goal of burning more calories than you take in, and how the food content (the macros) will help you maintain your health. The most important thing for patients is to determine their caloric needs to maintain their bodies and the percentages of macros they need to take in to sustain a healthy lifestyle. It's not easy to do that, but there's plenty of help today, whether it's using a program or an app and/or consulting with a nutritionist or specialist. It's crucial to log your food so that you know what's coming in and going out. I learned for myself that if I don't track what I put into my mouth, it's too hard for me to maintain what I have. Again, in the end, it's calories in and calories out.

I guarantee that if you follow a good food and fitness plan to the letter, and you're honest with yourself and log everything that you're putting into your mouth, you *will* lose weight.

STRESS REDUCTION

I mentioned in the previous chapter how moms are goers and doers and feel guilty about relaxing after surgery. It's important after surgery for moms to separate themselves for a short time from the stress of making lunches, picking the kids up and dropping them off at school and activities, and doing all the other goers-and-doers stuff. Reducing your stress is a good thing for anyone at any time, actually, and not just after surgery.

I get it that moms have to take care of their kids, it's innate. They can't separate themselves from it. But I can't tell you how many times patients will call me and say something like, "Oh, recovery's been so tough." I ask them to tell me what's going on. "It's all the stuff with the kids and my husband's working, and my breasts still really hurt." I point out that they're not really taking the time they need to recover, that they have to somehow step out of mommy mode a bit more than they're doing, if they're doing it at all. I suggest asking other people for help, even though we know moms have a hard time asking other people for help. Or they could ask their own older kids to step up and help. Their recovery isn't going well, because they're not getting rest and going to bed on time, and they're not avoiding stress. I truly believe that the mind and the body work together. If you're tired, you don't feel good, and you're not going to heal as well.

For the first four to six weeks or so after surgery, patients really need to step back and not be so much of a doer.

Now, carry that forward by finding ways to take breaks for yourself to unwind, relax, and let your stress go. Take a yoga or tai chi class, take a long walk, just sit quietly with your own thoughts and breathe, read a book, listen to music—these are some things that can help you break out of the goer-and-doer mode and just de-stress a bit. It's good for your heart, your mind, and your overall health, and it's really important not to feel guilty about doing it.

The new you means the whole person—not just how great you look after your surgery, but how you feel physically and mentally, and how you feel about yourself. You spent money, time, and energy for a good surgical procedure, and you had a good outcome. You might have lost some weight before surgery, and then you ate well and stayed fit afterward to maintain your results. The "new you" lifestyle is you just continuing these good habits, not for a few months or even a few years, but for the rest of your life.

CONCLUSION

Shortly before writing this, I performed a breast-augmentation surgery for a woman that resulted in an incredible transformation. She had lost 150 pounds prior to the surgery, but felt miserable in her skin, because her breasts were saggy, and she just didn't feel sexy. She was very uncomfortable in the bedroom with her husband. But just a breast augmentation literally changed her life. She didn't even need a lift. She's a completely different person now, just beaming with confidence, so cheerful about feeling like herself again—the way she always imagined she should feel after having had children and being a mom. Now she's completely confident in the bedroom without her clothes, whereas before the surgery, she didn't even want to take her clothes off. She still wanted a tummy tuck, but it's so amazing how just the breast augmentation made her feel like a new person.

In another recent case, I performed a breast augmentation, tummy tuck, and arm lift for another woman who'd had a massive weight loss. Clearly, these are life-defining moments for these people. After surgery, they feel like they've totally regained their lives and the ability to function in the world. When they're out and about in normal clothing, they feel like everyone's staring at them—not for bad reasons this time, but because they look so terrific, and how they feel about themselves inside again shows through, too. You can see it in the way they carry themselves. I see that change while it's happening, from the consultation to the preoperative visit to having the surgery and afterward, and just seeing the difference in their personas through all of those stages is quite compelling. I love that I can experience those kinds of changes in people's lives.

My Mommy Makeover patients are some of the best examples of cosmetic body rebuilding. Women who come in for Mommy Makeovers tend to lose their self-confidence completely after having children. The Mommy Makeover procedures give that confidence back to them, and more.

Happy wives aren't the only ones who make me smile. I see a lot of happy husbands, too. They come in with their wives and are just so supportive. They just want their wives to be happy and to feel good. When the husband's completely in favor of the surgery, you know that it's not about the money. When his wife feels better about herself, it can change their marriage.

That's my goal in all my cases. People come to me to feel and look like a new person, or to look more like their old selves before kids and gravity and the years started to take their toll—and plastic surgery can make it happen. If you want that kind of change in your life, you now have the tools and the information to find the right surgeon for you and get the body you want.

OUR SERVICES

Face Procedures: Facelift, necklift, fat transfer, eyebrow lift, upper- and lower-eyelid rejuvenation, chin augmentation

Breast: Breast augmentation, breast reduction, breast augmentation and lift, breast lift, breast-cancer reconstruction, nipple and areolar procedures, gynecomastia reduction (for men)

Body: Arm lift, thigh lift, abdominoplasty, liposuction, gluteal lift, gluteal augmentation with fat (Brazilian Butt Lift), or Sculptra injections

Spa Services: Neurotoxins (Botox), filler, face peels, dermabrasion, facials, laser treatments, microneedling, PRP (Platelet Rich Plasma) injections, hair restoration, non-surgical facial lifting, skin care, fat freezing, skin tightening

BROWN PLASTIC SURGERY
11000 N. Scottsdale Rd, Ste 100
Scottsdale, AZ 85254
480-947-2455

rbrown@rbrownmd.com
office@rbrownmd.com

www.richardjbrownmd.com